MEETING THE
LEADERSHIP
CHALLENGE
IN
LONG-TERM CARE

MEETING THE LEADERSHIP CHALLENGE
IN
LONG-TERM CARE

What You Do Matters

by

David Farrell, M.S.W., L.N.H.A.

Cathie Brady, M.S.

Barbara Frank, M.P.A.

Foreword by

V. Tellis-Nayak, Ph.D.

Mary Tellis-Nayak, R.N., M.S.N., M.P.H.

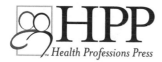

Health Professions Press

Baltimore • London • Sydney

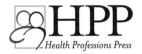

Health Professions Press, Inc.
Post Office Box 10624
Baltimore, Maryland 21285-0624

www.healthpropress.com

Interior design by Mindy Dunn and cover design by Erin Geoghegan.
Typeset by Blue Heron Typesetting.
Manufactured in the United States of America by Versa Press, East Peoria, Illinois.

This book is sold without warranties of any kind, express or implied, and the publisher and author disclaim any liability, loss, or damage caused by the contents of this book.

Continuing education units (CEUs) are available for long-term care administrators and nurses. Visit www.achca.org/ or call 202-536-5120 for more information.

Library of Congress Cataloging-in-Publication Data

Farrell, David, 1963-
   Meeting the leadership challenge in long-term care : what you do matters / by David Farrell, Cathie Brady, Barbara Frank.
      p. ; cm.
   Includes index.
   ISBN 978-1-932529-70-8 (pbk.)
   1. Long-term care facilities—Personnel management. 2. Nursing homes—Administration. 3. Leadership. I. Brady, Cathie, 1954– II. Frank, Barbara, 1955– III. Title.
   [DNLM: 1. Long-Term Care—organization & administration. 2. Health Services Administration. 3. Leadership. WX 162]
   RA999.A35F37 2011
   362.16068—dc22   2011003679

British Library Cataloguing in Publication data are available from the British Library.

To Susan Eaton

Her insightful research enlightened the field of long-term care.
With her genuine warmth toward people who work in
long-term care and her brilliance in identifying and sharing
good practices, she broke new ground and helped us all
understand *what a difference management makes!*
She inspired each of us—our shared appreciation of her
brought us together.

We are indebted to her and miss her dearly.

CONTENTS

ABOUT THE AUTHORS

David Farrell, M.S.W., L.N.H.A., has served as a licensed nursing home administrator in the long-term care profession for 25 years. He started as a certified nursing assistant while attending college and the experience inspired him to pursue a master's degree in social work with a concentration in gerontology and administration from Boston College. He has also focused on the importance of collecting data and sharing it with staff to determine needed improvements. As a nationally known leader in quality improvement and culture change, Farrell has documented the business case for providing a positive work environment and translated research about good leadership into daily practice. A published author and member of the Board of Directors at the Pioneer Network, he has delivered inspiring presentations to long-term care leaders at state conferences and corporate training events in nearly every state. While working for state Quality Improvement Organizations, he played a lead role in the National Nursing Home Quality Initiative. Farrell also served on the faculty team for the national Improving the Nursing Home Culture project involving QIOs and national nursing home corporations in 21 states. He has advised the Centers for Medicare and Medicaid Services on quality improvement and culture change. Currently, Farrell is Director of Organizational Development and Regional Director of Operations for a private nursing home management firm in California.

Cathie Brady, M.S., has more than 30 years of experience providing services and advocating for older adults in a variety of settings, including serving as Executive Director of the Department of Aging Services for the city of Bristol, Connecticut, and for 10 years as the Regional LTC Ombudsman for eastern Connecticut. Brady has an M.S. in Organizational Management from Eastern Connecticut State University. As co-founder (with co-author, Barbara Frank) of B&F Consulting, she facilitates nursing home improvements by developing leaders' abilities to nurture their staff and help people work better together. She served as faculty for a national 22-state pilot with Quality Partners of Rhode Island on Improving the Nursing Home Culture and co-produced a four-part Web cast series for the Center for Medicare and Medicaid

Services entitled "From Institutional to Individualized Care." Brady has directed several initiatives in Connecticut, Massachusetts, and Maine to support workplace learning and culture change and she co-developed a curriculum for Nurses as Mentors for a Robert Wood Johnson–funded Jobs to Careers initiative in Connecticut. For 3 years, she worked with the New Orleans Nursing Home Staffing Project, which helped nursing homes recover from the aftermath of Hurricane Katrina, and co-produced a film with Louisiana Public Broadcasting called *The Big Uneasy: Katrina's Unsung Heroes*. A frequent speaker at state and national conferences, Brady specializes in working with leaders who have the right instincts but who are overwhelmed by the challenges of being in nursing homes in need, special-focus facilities, critical access nursing homes, or otherwise challenged care organizations.

Barbara Frank, M.P.A., began her career working for 16 years at the National Citizens' Coalition for Nursing Home Reform in Washington, D.C., where she directed the landmark 1985 study "A Consumer Perspective on Quality Care: The Residents' Point of View" and helped establish the national network of state and local ombudsman programs. She facilitated the Campaign for Quality, through which providers, consumers, practitioners, and regulators developed consensus on what became the OBRA 1987 legislation that refocused nursing home regulations on individualized care. Frank facilitated the first Pioneer Network gathering in 1997, and in 2005 she facilitated the St. Louis Accord, a national gathering of providers, consumers, regulators, and quality improvement organizations that came together to improve clinical outcomes through staff stability and culture change. Co-founder (with her colleague and co-author, Cathie Brady) of B&F Consulting, she works directly with individual nursing homes to improve their stability, care outcomes, and quality of life. As faculty to the Quality Partners of Rhode Island Improving the Nursing Home Culture pilot, she helped 254 nursing homes improve staff, resident, and organizational outcomes, and co-produced Quality Partners' Staff Stability Toolkit and the four-part CMS Web series "From Institutional to Individualized Care." Frank also led a team in the New Orleans Nursing Home Staffing Project, which helped nursing homes recover from the aftermath of Hurricane Katrina. Frank co-produced a film with Louisiana Public Broadcasting called *The Big Uneasy: Katrina's Unsung Heroes*. She co-authored *Nursing Homes: Getting Good Care There* (1996). Frank serves on the board of the Pioneer Network and has a master's degree in public administration from the Kennedy School of Government.

ACKNOWLEDGMENTS

People matter the most! The authors would like to express deep gratitude to the many people who helped make this book a reality.

We are very grateful to Mary Jane Koren, M.D., M.P.H., Vice President for the Picker/Commonwealth Fund Long-Term Care Quality Improvement Program, and Lucile Hanscom, Executive Director of Picker Institute, for funding us to write this book through a grant to the American College of Health Care Administrators. Dr. Koren and Ms. Hanscom, and their respective foundations, are true champions of quality, person-centered long-term care. Their belief in our work and steadfast support were pivotal in giving us the ability to complete the book.

We thank Marianna Grachek, CEO of the American College of Health Care Administrators, for facilitating the grant process and providing professional review of this book by members and associates of ACHCA. Her ongoing support and the thoughtful feedback from her network helped us to make this a better book.

Quality Partners of Rhode Island deserves special recognition. The authors worked as a team with Dr. David Gifford, Gail Patry, Marguerite McLaughlin, and the staff at QPRI for Improving the Nursing Home Culture, a 2004–2005 pilot funded by the Centers for Medicare and Medicaid Services (CMS) involving 254 nursing homes. Many of the ideas reflected in this book grew from this work and were further formulated through our work with Quality Partners on the Staff Stability Toolkit, on the four-part CMS Webcast series "From Institutional to Individualized Care," and on the 9th Scope of Work with Nursing Homes in Need. With Quality Partners, we all developed a change process called the Holistic Approach to Transformational Change (HATCh), which recognizes the importance of workplace and leadership practices as the foundation for staff stability, individualized care, and quality improvement. Gail and Margie have been trusted friends, brilliant colleagues, and passionate contributors to the thoughts reflected in this book. We thank Quality Partners of Rhode Island for giving us the opportunity to develop materials and the continued support they have given us over the past years. And we thank Dr. Gifford for teaching us about spread.

We thank David Johnson, from IPRO (New York state's QIO), who meticulously developed the original drill-down tools from working drafts into their current form in the Staff Stability Toolkit. With an acute sensitivity to providers' needs, he shaped them into Excel spreadsheets that are easy to use and can be customized to each provider's unique circumstances.

We would also like to acknowledge the contribution of the many outstanding leaders in long-term care who have been our mentors and guides and whose valuable information is captured and shared in stories in this book. Many lessons and examples used in our book came from providers participating in the Critical Access Nursing Homes Initiative of Advancing Excellence in America's Nursing Homes Campaign; Better Jobs, Better Care–VT operated by Community of Vermont Elders (COVE); Connecticut CNA Advancement and Work-based Learning Initiatives operated by Capital Workforce Partners; Connecticut's Culture Change and Career Ladder Initiative operated by the 1199 Training and Upgrading Fund through the Connecticut Women's Education and Legal Fund; the Louisiana Workforce Initiative, including the New Orleans and Lake Charles Nursing Home Staffing Projects; the Massachusetts Extended Care Career Ladder Initiative operated by the Commonwealth Corporation; and the Quality Partners of Rhode Island Improving the Nursing Home Culture Pilot and the 9th Scope of Work Nursing Home in Need program.

In particular, we thank Lori Brothers, Sue Fortin, Sandy Godfrey, Bill Graves, Susan Hawver, Connie McDonald, Loren Salvietti, Lori Todd, and Scott West for allowing us to use examples from their experiences and for being role models of the leadership qualities we share in this book. We owe a special debt of gratitude to Lori Brothers, an administrator who, as she turned around a troubled facility, was a touchstone throughout the writing of this book. Her careful and candid reading of every chapter provided a reality check that the contents were helpful and relevant and an accurate reflection of her own home's 1-year journey from "special focus facility" to high performer.

We are grateful to those who read, edited, and cheered us on: Linda Sadden, Elise Nakhnikian, Sarah Burger, and Joseph Brady.

We are also grateful to Kate O'Malley and the California Health Care Foundation for funding the assessment of David Farrell's nursing home using the Artifacts for Culture Change tool developed by Karen Schoenemen and Carmen Bowman, and to Lois Cutler and Rosalie Kane for their ideas regarding how to improve the physical environment of nursing homes on a tight budget, which Farrell has also used.

As active members of the Pioneer Network, the authors thank its founders, leadership, participants, and staff for being beacons of individualized care and caring workplace practices. Special thanks to Barry Barkan, Charlene Boyd, Rose Marie Fagan, Joanne Rader, Bill Thomas, and Carter Williams for bringing their ideas and practices forward and nurturing the birth and growth of a movement for their widespread adoption. We thank Bonnie Kantor and Megan Hannan, who have provided extraordinary leadership to the Pioneer Network.

We thank the Centers for Medicare and Medicaid Services for funding the state Quality Improvement Organizations to assist nursing homes in improving quality and for their active engagement and support of Advancing Excellence, an incredible national collaboration. We also thank the Institute for Healthcare Improvement and the Breakthrough Series Collaborative Model for providing a valuable framework that has guided our work.

We acknowledge the National Citizens' Coalition for Nursing Home Reform (NCCNHR), now the National Consumer Voice for Quality Long-Term Care, for steadfast advocacy for high-quality individualized care, for facilitating the collaborative advocacy that brought us OBRA '87, and for shining a light on positive provider practices. Special thanks to Elma Holder, who founded the organization and whose steadfast vision for and commitment to good caring for older adults profoundly and positively shaped the nursing home field.

We thank V. Tellis-Nayak and Mary Tellis-Nayak for contributing their wisdom to the field throughout the years as well as for their foreword to the book.

We are grateful to Susan Eaton for her groundbreaking work, which we rely on in this book and for which we dedicate this book in her name.

We thank our publisher, Mary Magnus, and the team at Health Professions Press for guiding us through this process in a way that has honored the spirit of our work and helped us be our best.

Lastly, from David: A special thanks to my wife Brenda, the love of my life, and to my parents, Richard and Nancy, the most generous and caring people I know. Thank you for all of your love and support.

The Touchstone of Nursing Home Quality

Managers' Concerns for the Caregiver

Directors of nursing (DONs) and nursing home administrators (NHAs) across the United States are the unseen, hands-on leaders who mentor 1.3 million workers in the art of caring for older adults. This book speaks primarily to them and to their regional managers. It speaks as well to the unit leaders, supervisors, and activity coordinators who work under them. This book salutes these stalwarts for their remarkable contribution to the lives of our aging spouses, parents, and grandparents, and thereby for enhancing the quality of all our lives.

The authors counsel us with the authority and sensitivity born of the more than 75 combined years they have toiled in long-term care. They have served on national panels, addressed audiences across the U.S., counseled regulators, and shaped policy. They have left a trail of wise practices and sensible systems in their wake. In this book, they present profound ideas in commonsense language and distill their wisdom in real case studies.

The central theme of the book is the challenge long-term care poses to managers, the response it elicits from them, and why that response matters. The book examines how nursing home managers relate to their staff, in general, and to certified nursing assistants (CNAs), in particular—which are the defining measures of whether a nursing home is set on a sure path to success or on a road to nowhere.

An Improbable Community and Its Challenge to Managers

A nursing home is an improbable community unlike any other natural or planned community. It is an artificial creation held together by an uneasy coalition of interests: for-profit, service-minded, religious, and governmental. Often, the group starts as an assortment of individuals whose only common denominator is old age, frailty, and dependence. The staff that serve them differ markedly in age, race, ethnicity, culture, social class, and even nationality.

Nevertheless, we expect a nursing home to transcend these divisions and to achieve a person-centered community. To their great credit, many nursing homes have transformed themselves into stable, person-centered communities where residents and staff stay connected in warm friendship. This is indeed a singular achievement, although we rarely publicly acclaim the feat.

The ground zero of this unusual transformation is the precarious encounter between a CNA and a resident—two parties with unlike backgrounds, both belonging to groups that are socially the most powerless and the least esteemed, and who spend significant hours each day in close and even intimate contact. It is in the chemistry of their uncertain interchange that nursing home quality germinates and sprouts to life.

The expert hands that solicitously tend that nascent quality, guide its growth, and nurture it into maturity are the DON and the NHA. (We will refer to this team as *managers*.) As managers, they have to build resident–staff trust across social gaps. They have to heal the trauma of residents freshly uprooted from their familiar world and shaken by the thought that they will live their last years under one roof with strangers. They have to address the anxieties, needs, and desires of both the residents and staff. Above all, they have to create policy, to design protocols, and to foster care practices—the platform that supports the budding community of trust.

A tall order! Across the United States, about 34,000 brave DONs and NHAs have accepted this awesome responsibility. They mentor 650,000 CNAs, 130,000 registered nurses (RNs), 185,000 licensed practical nurses (LPNs), and 400,000 other staff in the art of adding quality to the life of nursing home residents. In 17,000 nursing homes, they direct real-life dramas of idealism, selflessness, and dedication that edify and inspire. These everyday heroes do not make the headlines, nor do they get the pat on the back they deserve. Too much fog impedes the public's grasp of the day-to-day life and achievements inside the walls of nursing homes.

Turnover: The Bane of Long-term Care

Worse than public ignorance, are the dogma and prejudice that creep into professional dialogue, slant policy, and misguide practice. Social figments have always permeated all aspects of modern healthcare, but nowhere more so than in long-term care, nowhere as negatively as in nursing home care, and not with as formidable an impact as in matters affecting caregivers. Management manuals and workshops unwittingly perpetuate biased theories, giving legitimacy to faulty management practices and unsound personnel policies that impede and misguide well-meaning managers.

CNA turnover, a pivotal issue for many nursing homes, is an apt example. We still do not agree on what forces singly or cumulatively aggravate or reduce turnover. Many managers are ill informed, misinformed, confused, or frustrated by the layers of myth, bias, and bad advice that obscure the subject of CNA turnover.

CNA turnover is the bane of too many nursing homes. As CNAs leave in droves, money washes down the drain. Turnover burdens those CNAs who stay; it dents their morale. The upheaval adds insecurity to the life of residents. Rotating caregivers become less conversant with residents' personal and clinical needs. A heavy presence of agency-based temporary staff alters the tone of the workplace. Efficiency and competence rise in priority, impersonal care becomes the norm, and the CNA–resident bond is frowned upon.

These are legitimate concerns, but they should not gloss over the nuances in the turnover trends. Yes, the numbers are grim. In 2010, nearly 500,000 CNAs left their posts. Still, is all turnover bad? Many streams flow out of the nursing home, merge, and make up the flood of outward-bound CNAs. One stream results when nursing homes let the less devoted and unmotivated workers leave, voluntarily or not, thereby making room for fresh talent. Losing a loser is a gain, not a loss.

Another stream is often made up of college students, who neither lack motivation nor skill; but they never intended to stay. They work at a nursing home not as a first step on their chosen career path, but because the nursing home lets them temporarily supplement their meager finances at a convenient location and with a suitable work schedule.

A variant of the college-student type is a group of young and eager souls who are motivated by a vague sense of altruism and a desire to help people. They are not sure they want to make the commitment, yet they wish to test the waters. The stark demands of working in a nursing home soon take a toll on their spirit and idealism, and, wisely, many walk away.

Another outflowing stream that unduly inflates turnover statistics is the group of talented and motivated CNAs who have done a good job and are eager for a greater challenge. They move up in the profession and thereby enrich the supervisory and managerial ranks with their bedside experience. An overwhelming number of long-term care nurses who today serve in top executive and policy positions began their careers as CNAs. No one wishes to lower turnover rates by fencing in such talent desirous of promoting quality on a wider scale.

Turnover Virus Spares No Sector, Profession, or Position

The 2010 report by the American Health Care Association (AHCA) of a sample of over 2,000 nursing homes surveyed in 2008 estimated the prevalence of turnover and retention. The 17,000 nursing homes nationwide hire more than 1 million workers, 65% of whom provide nursing services. Well over three quarters of a million of these nursing workers (more than 60%) are CNAs.[3]

The CNA turnover rate for 2008 stood at 54%. Many close observers of the field have concluded that the CNA turnover rate nationwide steadily declined through 2010. Turnover in 2008 was 43% among LPNs and 43% among RNs. The study also found that the turnover rate for administrators was 23% and 18% for DONs. The AHCA's 2002 survey had reported a 49.7% turnover rate for DONs that ranged at the state level from 14.8% to 142.7%, with 5.8% of positions vacant.[2] Another study reported that in the early 2000s more than 7,000 NHAs left their jobs each year, and that in recent years the rate had been above 40%.[7]

Two studies concluded that turnover in the ranks of managers is a paradox.[6,7] First, DONs and NHAs love their profession and find their roles satisfying. Second, regulation and the threat of lawsuits have redefined their roles and have made them part compliance officer, part traffic cop, and part paper-pushing bureaucrat. Managers do not relish these new roles, more so because they have had no training in them. They especially resent these obligations because they deny managers the joy of caring and mentoring—what drew them to long-term care in the first place. Satisfied managers, when frustrated and alienated, head toward the exit door.

Research has confirmed what close observers have long believed: stable managers are the foundation of good quality in long-term care. Their turnover triggers a cascading effect: staff morale drops, staff turnover rises, care systems come apart, caregiving suffers, state survey results worsen, satisfaction among staff and families declines, and census falls. Persistent manager turnover, in sum, portends a meltdown in quality.([6, 7])

There is a lesson to be learned from a turnover epidemic in which 43% of workers walk out every year. The turnover virus spares no economic sector; it infects some sectors worse than it does nursing homes; it spares no high-status profession or high-income position.([1, 5, 9]) In other words, the offer of higher wages and higher status may not be sufficient incentives to stem the turnover tide. Turnover among CNAs illustrates this point.

The work of CNAs is often described as menial and CNAs are remunerated at about minimum wage. CNA turnover, however, follows an unexpected pattern. Amid high CNA turnover, a solid core of them stays on, creating stability and ensuring continuity of care and relationships. Researchers at My InnerView studied stability in 293 nursing homes and learned that 12% of the 4,452 CNAs employed by homes had quit within 3 months of their start day, whereas a solid 70% had served in the same facility for more than a year, 15% had served for 5 to 10 years, and another 15% had served for more than 10 years.([8])

Workplace Quality Affects Quality of Life

Researchers wanting to know what contributes to CNA commitment and what breeds CNA alienation surveyed CNAs in 156 nursing homes to see how their work environment influenced their commitment to stay.([7]) The study defined work environment as the workplace atmosphere engendered by nine elements: workplace safety, adequate tools to do a good job, fair evaluations, reasonable wages, intrinsic reward of one's work, help dealing with job stress, inter-shift communication, staff team spirit, and staff respect for residents.

The study found that nothing affects a CNA's commitment as much as does her work setting, and no one stirs a CNA as much as the managers do. A CNA spends half of her waking hours at the nursing home, which is the source of her income, work identity, and relationships outside the home. The impact that managers exert on the CNA is potent, primal, and pervasive; it reaches beyond her work life and into her personal life. The quality of her workplace greatly determines the quality of her life.

CNAs rate their work environment almost exactly how they rate their managers. In other words, CNAs view their work environment as an extension of their managers' concern for them. The work setting is the direct handiwork of their managers; it bears their signature; it reflects their values, priorities, and interests. It is a sure measure of how managers view the CNAs, how much they value and care about them.

The study found that low pay and heavy workloads cause stress for CNAs, and that CNAs find joy when they feel their work makes a difference. CNAs who are satisfied with managers, however, show less dissatisfaction with their pay and workloads, and find their work more rewarding. That is, good managers increase satisfaction across the board, and not so good managers increase widespread dissatisfaction.

What precisely do good managers do to win over CNAs and why do mediocre ones sour them? Good managers look at CNAs in two ways that are very different from the way that not-so-good managers do. First, good managers look upon a CNA as a person with intrinsic value, and, second, they do not consider that a CNA's social origin diminishes her intrinsic value as a person.

The Touchstone of Quality: Managers' Mindset

Social science rests on an axiom: We do not see life in its fullness. Unknowingly we filter the human element out of work and workers, and view them primarily in economic terms. Our language, tradition, law, and custom all encourage the belief that life is competitive, everything has a cost, self-interest is the engine of progress. In employer–employee relations, rules of economics should be our guide. Emotions, relationships, altruism, and morality should not interfere with the workings of the economic model.

Many of us also carry a second mental template. This tendency distorts a manager's view of workers such as CNAs. When you as a manager meet a CNA, your mind first alerts you not to the CNA, *the person*, but *the CNA*, an individual lower than you in status, with a humble background and lacking middle class values, virtues, and work ethic.

Unwittingly and innocently, these distorted ways of thinking affect our everyday speech and action. Our well-meaning use of words such as *labor market, work force, human resource, staffing ratio, facility, bed count, occupancy,* or *probationary period* show how much we have embraced this prevalent mindset. Notice how readily we use such words when we speak of those at the bottom of the corporate pyramid and how rarely when referring to those who lord over it. When using such language, without perhaps realizing it, we subtly diminish the humanity of the residents and of the caregivers.

In personnel relations, we studiously stay clear of vocabulary that refers to the most human emotions: *affection, fondness, charity, compassion, devotion, mercy, intimacy, tenderness,* and *love*—all linked to healing relationships. We measure *satisfaction*, but not *happiness, joy* and *friendship*, which are truer indicators of quality outcomes. We calculate *staffing ratios*, but pretend we cannot compute the more apt *ratios of compassionate approach and devoted care*. Was Einstein right: "Not everything that counts is countable, and not everything that's countable counts"?

Unconscious biases, law, language, and professional protocol all bear upon nursing home managers and urge them to see the CNA through a mental lens that blurs out the real, human person in the CNA role, and presents her as a mere cog in the business of running the nursing home enterprise. This point of view justifies why the manager should not be distracted by the CNA's personal troubles and private affairs.

This book upholds a very different type of an exemplary manager, one who casts aside these blinders and connects directly with the breathing and feeling person hidden behind this social fiction. Great managers have the ability (be it an innate gift or a cultivated skill) to recognize and relate to the human being inside everyone they deal with—inside the failing bodies of their residents, behind the unsophisticated behaviors of some staff, and beneath the distress of the visiting family. They understand that each person is unique in makeup, yet no different from anyone else in the universal human need to be valued.

This is the litmus test of nursing home quality, as the authors see it. If nursing home managers genuinely honor and value the CNA as they would every person regardless of rank and authority, then their nursing home is assuredly set firmly on the right path to the desired end. The authors lay out the path and the signposts that would undoubtedly help such nursing homes to reach the goal.

Conversely, managers who look at life with eyes jaundiced by the prevalent mindset put their nursing home on a perilous course. They orient it in a direction away from their desired terminus. They doom every quality initiative to failure. Hoping to reach the goal of person-centered care with this mistaken mindset is an absurd contradiction.

This book is an antidote to this all too common mindset. It urges managers to heed the yearnings in their own heart—the need to be respected, the desire to belong, and the urge to transcend and to give. Those very longings also seek fulfillment within a CNA. Good managers offer the CNA all the tools and support she needs. They set her up for success; they give her room to grow, to express her talent, and to create; they ensure that residents take notice and applaud her success; they create settings in which informal encounters grow into friendships. Like an engineer, they tweak care processes, tinker with systems, and marshal all resources to attain the goals they have set. Like a bandleader, they motivate and persuade those out of tune and bring nursing home life into harmony with the themes of a person-centered community.

Good managers empathize with the CNA who shows up at work, but who is unable to leave her private anxieties at the doorstep. Her troubles follow her to the residents' bedsides, and workday aggravations make them seem heavier. Her unit is short-staffed. She smarts when her supervisor reproaches her in front of visitors. A resident's son is annoyed with the administrator and takes it out on her. She winces as the half-confused 88-year-old again spits out a racial epithet.

The CNA notices that good managers anticipate and effectively act to prevent the daily irritants that assault her self-image and self-worth. She soon learns that the character and quality of her work environment reflect how the managers perceive her, value her, and care for her as a person. Good managers make the workplace a haven from private troubles and an environment that enriches quality of life.

The CNA in turn appreciates her managers, holds them in high esteem and readily gives them her loyalty. She will not fault them for the meager wages she takes home. She sleeps well at night thinking of the difference she makes in the lives of residents who depend on her, press her hand, and whisper "Thank you." Her troubles fade when she thinks of how residents' faces light up when she shows up for work. She will not give up these deeply spiritual rewards for just a few more pennies an hour, or maybe not even for a fortune. A fun and rewarding workplace, co-worker camaraderie, a bond with residents, and feelings of responsibility to managers to whom she can always turn when in need, all these evoke a commitment from her that transcends mere economic calculus.

Managers execute a wondrous feat with the elders and staff who, like marbles in a box, live in close contact without relating to each other. In Part I of this book, David Farrell's journal illustrates how with imagination and persuasion managers replace that emotional isolation with an interpersonal chemistry of mutual esteem and trust. Managers create the precise conditions that make that chemistry spread and give rise to a caring, person-centered culture in which CNAs are committed and residents are happy.

Transforming staff into devoted caregivers is the single challenge, among thousands, that tests the humanity and moral fiber of the manager. No reward or sanction on its own will elicit staff commitment. Only a safe, supportive, and satisfying work environment—the only true proof of the managers' genuine concern—will persuade staff to give the manager unwavering loyalty, and will motivate them to walk the extra mile for the residents.(4) When managers win this first and decisive battle, they have, in effect, won the war and have set their nursing home firmly on the path toward being a loving, person-centered community.

In *Meeting the Leadership Challenge in Long-Term Care*, the authors generously share their winning recipes, proven strategies, and tested programs, drawn from their rich experiences. Their passion will inspire you to meet the leadership challenge and to speed your progress toward the shared ideal we all seek.

What you do matters—greatly!

V. Tellis-Nayak, Ph.D.
Mary Tellis-Nayak, R.N., M.S.N., M.P.H.
Chicago, Illinois

Notes

1. American Association of Colleges of Nursing. (2010). Fact Sheet.

2. American Health Care Association. (2003). "Results of the 2002 AHCA survey of nursing staff vacancy and turnover in nursing homes," pp. 14–15. Available at http://www.ahca.org/research/rpt_vts2002_final.pdf.

3. American Health Care Association. (2010). "Report of findings: 2008 survey of nursing staff vacancy and turnover in nursing facilities."

4. McGlothlin, Jr., C. W., & Streetman, A. B. (2009, Spring). "Analysis of Ergonomic-Related Injuries in Nursing Homes: A Case Study." *Journal of SH&E Research*, Feature Article 7, American Society of Safety Engineers.

5. Malloch, K., & Porter-O'Grady, T. (2009). "The quantum leader: Applications for the new world of work." PricewaterhouseCoopers' Health Research Institute.

6. Tellis-Nayak, V. (2005). "Who will care for the caregivers?" *Health Progress*, 86(6):37–43.

7. Tellis-Nayak, V. (2007). The Satisfied but disenchanted leaders in long-term care: The paradox of the nursing home administrator. *Seniors Housing & Care Journal*, 15(1):3–18.

8. Tellis-Nayak, V. (2007). "CNA turnover and stability." My InnerView, Wausau, WI.

9. U.S. Department of Labor, Bureau of Labor Statistics. (2010). "Hires and separation rates, government and private industry, June 2010." Available at http://www.bls.gov/opub/ted/2010/ted_20100816.htm.

A NOTE TO OUR READERS

"Buddy, I feel your pain."

With those words David Farrell joined Barbara Frank and Cathie Brady in helping Scott West get a handle on the turnover that was destabilizing his nursing home as part of an initiative called Better Jobs, Better Care (BJBC). As administrator of Birchwood Terrace Healthcare, West had been working so hard to deal with the everyday crises that came from having to plug holes in each shift's schedule that he had not been able to step back to get a handle on what he could do to stop the vicious cycle of instability. His challenges were not unique; nor were the ways he was trying to deal with them. The industry norms just were not working. Like so many others, West was paying bonuses to people who would fill in at the last minute rather than rewarding his steady staff for their dependability. When he stepped back to look at the situation, he saw he was spending over $1 million a year on the causes and effects of turnover and less than one-tenth that amount on interventions and rewards to support the existing staff in their work. Collecting data and analyzing the root cause of his problems eventually allowed West to make the case to his regional corporate vice president to spend smarter by rewarding reliability. As his efforts started to pay off, he concentrated on developing the leadership skills of his management team. Together these changes produced sustained stability.

There is no reason why other nursing home leaders can't enjoy the same rewards in their own communities. We have written this book to help show the way.

What a difference management makes!

We three first met at the 2004 Pioneer Network conference, drawn together by our mutual appreciation of Susan Eaton's "What a difference management makes!" (see A Note About Our Sources at end of book). We'd each found Eaton's work compelling and foundational, especially her description of the "vicious cycle" in homes with high turnover, and the practices she consistently found in place in homes with low turnover. Our appreciation for her work was only the beginning of what we found we have in common.

We share a deep admiration for the courageous and compassion-ate work of administrators, directors of nursing, and others who pro-vide leadership in nursing homes all over the country and who face the enormous challenges of providing long-term care services in an unforgiving, overbearing, and resource-depleted environment. We ap-plaud their dedication, sense of responsibility, spirit, and innovation in providing care to frail elders. We want to support their professional growth by sharing the good practices that we have learned through our work with nursing home leaders across the country. We know sharing these practices will improve leaders' abilities to do their work and con-sequently improve the lives of residents in their care.

This book is a synthesis of what we have learned from our on-the-ground experiences all over the country. Farrell has worked as an administrator, Quality Improvement Organization (QIO) consultant, and corporate regional staff member. Brady and Frank first as advocates, and then as co-founders of B&F Consulting, have worked directly with nursing homes and in collaboration with QIOs, workforce develop-ment networks, culture change coalitions, and other state initiatives.

Workforce First

We first formally collaborated through a Centers for Medicare and Medicaid Services–funded (CMS) pilot in 2004–2005 called Improv-ing the Nursing Home Culture (INHC). The study was conducted by Quality Partners of Rhode Island, led by Marguerite McLaughlin, Gail Patry, and David Gifford. We were the faculty for the pilot, Farrell, as a Quality Partners staff member; and Frank and Brady, as subcontractors. It involved 254 nursing homes in 21 states and was designed to help the homes improve staff retention and individualize care for residents. In addition to lowering turnover, the participating homes succeeded in improving their clinical measures as a direct result of improvements in staff stability and individualized care.

The pilot used a model for change called the Holistic Approach to Transformational Change (HATCh; see figure). The HATCh model recognizes that resident care (represented by the heart in the middle of the figure) is always affected by the interplay of care practices, the physical environment, and workplace practices.

We used both the science and the psychology of change—inte-grating staff engagement into the quality improvement process. Con-nie McDonald, administrator at Maine General Rehabilitation and

The HATCh Model

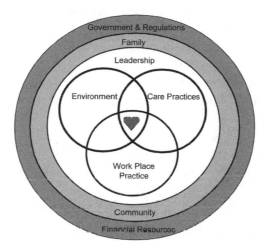

Nursing Care at Glenridge in Augusta, Maine, served as guest faculty to the pilot and participated with her staff in the film *Culture Change in Long-Term Care: A Case Study*, which served as an instructional resource for pilot participants. Her focus on staff stability, people development, and inclusion served as a guide for all the homes involved in the pilot. We helped participating nursing homes apply these practices immediately through "homework assignments" designed to help them discover what their staff and residents were experiencing and learn how to engage staff in working together to make improvements.

A major finding of the pilot was "workforce first"—the idea that staff stability and engagement was the prerequisite to being able to individualize care and improve clinically.

People Matter Most

In the closing session of the pilot, we asked participants to identify their most significant lessons. Participants concluded that people matter most. One corporate representative said he was struck by how much genuinely caring about and listening to his staff had been crucial to his company's success in achieving stability and clinical improvements. Others affirmed that the key ingredient to their success was paying attention to what staff needed and had to say.

Participants said they learned how to lead in a way that brought out the best in their staff. They said that while they as leaders had good ideas, their organizations benefited far more by tapping into the good ideas of all their staff and then "enabling them to act" to implement those ideas. This notion of enabling others to act came from Kouzes and Posner's *The Leadership Challenge*, a resource used in the pilot (see A Note About Our Sources).

Participants in the pilot also said they valued the opportunity to work collaboratively with each other. Having previously viewed each other as competitors, they had come to appreciate being able to "share shamelessly" their own innovations and challenges, and to learn from the experiences of their colleagues. We all saw the power of sharing and spreading the learning.

To Get Something Different, You Have To Do Something Different

Working with West at the same time as the pilot, we recognized the universality of West's experience and the wide applicability of the process he was using to achieve sustained stability. Drawing on examples from Birchwood, we developed homework assignments for the INHC participants to guide them in "drilling down" to examine how their own fiscal and management practices affected their turnover. Just as West had come to see how these "accepted" practices contributed to turnover, the homes in the pilot realized that getting different results required them to break from the industry norms and do something different. A BJBC case study capturing the work at Birchwood ultimately formed the basis for a Quality Partners Staff Stability Toolkit, available at www.qualitypartnersri.org. Also, Chapter 5, Achieving Staff Stability, is adapted from the case study. The Staff Stability Toolkit includes the drill-down tools used by West and the pilot participants, along with instructions on their use. For the toolkit, David Johnson, from IPRO (New York state's QIO), converted the original tools into their current form as Microsoft Excel spreadsheets that are easy to use and can be customized by each user (see the Appendixes).

What You Do Matters

Following these projects, Farrell returned to on-the-ground work as a nursing home administrator, putting what he had learned from the QIO world to use. In his previous work as an administrator, he had intuitively been successful through an approach that started with valuing and supporting his staff and then used basic QI principles to make change. He understood the value of data and what it could show about the impact that staff and management efforts were having. He decided to keep a journal to capture the realities of the day-to-day life of a nursing home administrator. He also kept a page of reminders on his desk to help ground himself when the pushes and pulls from corporate and regulatory overseers or the daily challenges of running the nursing home overwhelmed him. From time to time, Farrell would send off one of his late night journal entries to a small circle of colleagues and, with their encouragement, eventually started incorporating the entries into his public speaking engagements because of their power to portray the struggles and successes in this challenging work.

Meanwhile, Frank and Brady led an effort in the aftermath of Hurricane Katrina to support nursing homes in the New Orleans area that faced enormous staffing challenges after the storm's devastation. In collaboration with Susan Wehry, M.D., and Louisiana State Ombudsman Linda Sadden, they facilitated a process of mutual aid and collaboration among the 50 nursing homes in the affected area, working in partnership with the relevant state agencies and organizations. What New Orleans long-term care leaders did had a significant impact on their staff stability, even as the entire region was in disarray. For example, while every home struggled to find staff, some housed staff and their families whose own homes were destroyed by the post-Katrina floods. Staff told story after story about the impact their leaders' caring had on their own ability to recover personally and to sustain themselves through the hard times. Though we never conducted an official study of the recovery, the link between taking care of staff and taking care of residents became undeniable. We captured this experience and its lessons in *The Big Uneasy: Katrina's Unsung Heroes*, a video co-produced with Louisiana Public Broadcasting.

Despite the remarkable circumstances in New Orleans, Frank and Brady observed that the experiences of these nursing homes corresponded with those they'd repeatedly observed elsewhere through their work and investigations: in the homes researched by Eaton in "What a difference management makes!"; in the homes that participated in the Quality Partners pilot; at Birchwood Terrace, and in the experiences described in Farrell's journal. The common denominator was that what leaders do really matters to staff and resident well-being. This was the case even in New Orleans, where the enormous devastation faced by the area would seem to dominate the equation. What nursing home leaders did there had an enormous impact on staff's ability to work together in the face of intense adversity.

A Field Guide for Long-term Care Leaders

The idea of bringing all of this hard-won knowledge and experience together in a book that could serve as a guide to the field was embraced and funded by The Commonwealth Fund and the Picker Institute. Through grants to the American College of Health Care Administrators, The Commonwealth Fund and the Picker Institute supported our efforts to share these good management practices with administrators everywhere who want to make a positive difference.

This book captures our collective experiences from the trenches and in support of others who are working hands-on in the field of long-term care. This is not a research report; nor is it a comprehensive review of the literature or the field. Rather, it is a practical field guide to help administrators, directors of nursing, corporate regional staff, and other long-term care leaders put into practice the successful strategies we have learned along the way.

Moving the Flywheel

Jim Collins, in *Good to Great*, uses the analogy of "moving the flywheel" when describing the process of gaining momentum for positive change (see A Note About Our Sources). He describes the slow process at first to get the flywheel going, when each change is hard to accomplish because of all the ways an organization is burdened by systems, mindsets, and habits that have kept it in its current condition. As with a flywheel, each step in positive progress provides traction for acceleration. When the flywheel is in full swing, change can happen at an accelerated rate as the newly established circumstances become the new norm that contributes to further positive change. For example, when there is instability, it is difficult to sustain any new clinical protocols that have been put in place, and when a facility begins to achieve staff stability, it can get real traction for implementation of new practices because people are not strained by the stress of daily instability.

From the earliest implementations of our methods we have seen the flywheel effect. We have continued to hone our interventions so that we now know how to push the levers for positive change more quickly. Farrell took 9 months to turn around the home he writes about in his journal, but now as a corporate regional staff person he has been able to "cut to the chase" and get homes stabilized within a few short months. He focuses on supporting the people who are working well, bringing out the best in those who can step up, and replacing those few staff who drag down the organization. He cares about staff and makes sure they have the supplies, resources, and supports to do their jobs. He gives them the tools, skills, and information they need to make improvements. People consistently respond well to being trusted, heard, and supported.

Brady and Frank have similarly honed their interventions and seen homes quickly get traction for positive change by integrating staff engagement, individualized care, and quality improvement. Homes starting with stability are able to take their performance to another level through staff engagement in the change process. Homes facing significant challenges—homes identified as troubled by state survey directors and QIOs, homes in contentious union situations, resource-strapped homes, and homes entangled in large government bureaucracies—turn around quickly when they tune in to staff's needs and engage staff in working together for everyone's benefit. Lori Brothers, an administrator who turned around one such home, describes starting her transformation by caring about staff personally, making sure they had what they needed to do their jobs, and bringing them into committees she established to make the wholesale improvements necessary to provide good care.

In It Together

It doesn't take a natural disaster such as Hurricane Katrina to create a nursing home environment that fosters the atmosphere that everyone is "in this together." For nursing homes entangled in a vicious cycle of instability and demoralization this may seem like an oversimplified solution. The good news, however, is that being in it together really works, and can take you from contention to high performance in short order.

As Susan Hawver, administrator, was sharing information at a statewide conference about how her home made the journey from "nursing home in need to nursing home in the lead," she started her presentation by saying, "it's really all about being human and being caring; that's what made the difference in our organization." This is the universal answer. When staff know you care about them and have their back, they will respond in turn. When they trust you will listen to them and follow through on taking care of what they need to do their jobs, your organization will be well on its path to stability, good care, and strong organizational performance. One New Orleans administrator said, "They'll walk to the end of the earth for you if they feel like they're valued and they're respected. I think that's what helped us."

In every place we've worked the vivacity felt throughout the organization is palpable when staff from every corner step up to the challenge and opportunity of inclusion.

Eaton wrote:

> My relationships with hundreds of workers convinced me that work itself, no matter how low paid or "unskilled," is fundamental to most people's lives—not just in the sense of earning their livings, but in their own sense of who they are and what they are accomplishing in this world. . . . Most people have a sense of "making a difference" in the world through what they do, whether it is cleaning toilets, changing bandages, teaching others, or running a sewing machine. If they do not have such a sense, they yearn for it.
>
> Most people both want to do a good job and to make a difference through their labor. They hate not having the proper tools or training to complete their tasks. They hate not being asked how they might do their jobs better. And those who are not asked—which in my experience was especially true for those at the bottom of the workplace ladder—especially have a lot to contribute.

Staff everywhere are ready to be engaged—all you need do is invite them in, listen to what they have to say, and truly care about them. Working together, you'll be able to make your home a better place to live and work.

INTRODUCTION

What you do *does* matter. This book serves both as a wake-up call to leaders who doubt their impact and as an affirmation to leaders who vigorously take up the challenge each day of making the most of their impact. Based on the real-life experiences of the authors and other leaders in the field with whom they have worked, *Meeting the Leadership Challenge in Long-term Care* offers practical, commonsense, easy-to-implement practices that will yield immediate positive results. The book is constructed to allow readers to pick it up at any point, based on need and interest. Although the chapters are ultimately linked, they are also stand-alone.

Part I, Leadership, begins with journal entries from a year in the life of a nursing home administrator. David Farrell details his experiences turning around a home that was by all measures doing poorly. In a year's time, Farrell was able to stabilize staffing, improve quality, and generate profit. His journal is not your usual sanitized description; it is real, gritty, and inspiring. He depicts the difficulties, the triumphs, the tragedies, and the mundane. From painting over daily graffiti to reassuring distressed certified nursing assistants (CNAs) and residents, he captures how hard as well as rewarding being a long-term care administrator can be. Farrell's real-life experiences provide a blueprint for practices that any administrator can put in play. He cares deeply about his staff and his residents. By putting their interests first, he leads the organization to perform at its best.

Part I concludes with Chapter 1 which, building on Farrell's experiences, describes leadership practices that make a difference. Too often long-term care leaders are overwhelmed by regulatory and corporate oversight and feel the limits of what they can do more than the possibilities. For example, many leaders accept the common myth in long-term care that staff turnover is an inevitable cost of doing business. This chapter debunks that myth and the common practices that stem from it. The fact is that, time and again, administrators who take daily work life in hand in their nursing homes achieve stability. Chapter 1 provides a step-by-step field guide for leaders who want to make a positive difference.

In Part II, Practices for Stability, Chapters 2 and 3 detail concrete strategies for hiring the right people and promoting their attendance.

Chapter 2, Taking Time to Hire Right, includes methods for getting the right pool of candidates, screening well, and having a good welcoming process. Chapter 3, From Absenteeism to Attendance, describes ways to track and respond to absences, and support and reward good attendance.

Part II continues with Chapter 4, A Positive Chain of Leadership, which guides readers in how to provide the kind of daily supervision and leadership that bring out the best in staff. Chapter 4 describes how to make a difference in day-to-day supervision by developing the abilities of staff, modeling and promoting teamwork, and facilitating daily problem solving. Investing in your staff's development is how you invest in your organization.

Chapter 5, Achieving Staff Stability, is a case study that brings together all of the practices detailed in Part II. The chapter draws a link between management attention to staff needs and staff stability. It chronicles how leaders in one organization re-examined their fiscal and management practices and realized they were fueling their own instability by employing bonus practices common in the field—sign-on bonuses, bonuses for staff to take last-minute assignments—instead of rewarding staff who are reliable. The chapter describes how administrator Scott West used classic quality-improvement processes to analyze data, do root-cause analysis, and put in place effective fiscal and management practices to achieve sustained stability.

Part III, Moving the Flywheel, describes the *how* of change. It builds on the concept of gaining momentum for positive change as discussed in Jim Collins' book, *Good to Great* (see A Note About Our Sources at end of book). Chapter 6 provides the basics for an effective change process, and Chapter 7 focuses on how to get traction in your change efforts. Both chapters address how to integrate quality improvement (QI), individualized care, and workplace stability practices to support problem solving from the ground up. Staff stability and engagement are the prerequisites for high performance. While QI is often associated only with clinical initiatives, it is equally useful in examining the extent and root causes of instability and implementing successful interventions to achieve stability. Chapters 6 and 7 describe how to integrate the science and the psychology of QI, by using a high level of staff engagement in the change process.

Chapter 6 provides a step-by-step guide to high involvement. It cites leadership examples from a number of homes, including the extraordinary circumstances in New Orleans nursing homes during and after Hurricane Katrina. Leaders from these homes affirm the value of involving and listening to their staff in the decision-making process. Staff "let their minds go" and were able to innovate to address unprecedented challenges. The involvement continues post crisis and has contributed to many homes' ability to rebound from the devastation.

Chapter 7 describes structural processes to put in place to support good working relationships, including change-of-shift and start-of-shift meetings. It explains the importance of starting any change process by addressing causes of staff stress, because their areas of stress are usually the "canaries in the coal mine"—indicators of processes within the facility that are not working and rife with errors. Practices such as all hands on deck and managing by walking around help alleviate stress while building teamwork. When stressors are relieved, staff are free to work on making other improvements. Getting traction starts with engaging staff in efforts that bring immediate tangible benefits to them and to residents. The chapter suggests opportunities for changes in care practices that individualize care for residents while reducing staff stress.

The book concludes with Chapter 8, Memo to Corporate, in which we once again hear directly from David Farrell about practices that he, now as a corporate regional representative, has come to recognize he needs to put on his "Stop Doing List." It explains the negative impact of common practices, such as "drive-by consulting" and those endless demands for instant turnaround of data that reflect an expectation that administrators should be in their offices answering e-mails instead of making rounds out on the floor. The chapter offers specific suggestions for practices corporate staff can employ to make a positive difference in support of their on-site leadership.

Our book is not a comprehensive review of the literature. Nor is it the result of specific research. It is based on our direct experiences as well as those of people with whom we are in touch who work in nursing homes across the country.

This is a highly regulated field that quite often has only intrinsic rewards. *Meeting the Leadership Challenge in Long-term Care* highlights the deep caring and good practices that abound in this field. It is a vote of confidence to those who toil daily to care for others. What you do does matter! Your efforts make a difference. Make sure to make the most of them. We hope this book will help you along the way.

## PART I

Leadership

Journal

A Year in the Life of a Nursing Home Administrator

David J. Farrell

May 3, 2006

I arrived pretty early on my first day of orientation with the outgoing administrator. I anticipated that she might come in after 9:00, so I made it a point to be there at 7:30. I wanted to see the place wake up.

While orienting with the outgoing administrator, I was shocked that on at least three occasions, she referred to people working there as "the blacks." I wondered how she got away with saying that so freely, especially considering that white Anglo-Saxons like herself were clearly in the minority at this facility.

Her office was a mess. I noticed broken, shabby furniture in a small, crowded room that had been converted from a resident room. She had a sliding glass door but advised me not to open it "because the staff that work here are thieves and they would steal from this office if the room were left unattended." The vertical blinds were missing from the sliding glass door. She had no pictures on her walls. Her office looked similar to the whole facility—neglected.

In the afternoon of my third day of orientation, I was making rounds when I caught eyes with an African American resident who was sitting up in his bed. His was the third bed, by the window, in this three-bed room. I waved and he summoned me in.

As I walked into the room, I noticed the dingy linoleum tile floors, a large open closet without a door, and the glass in the windows, which appeared to be dirty. As I got closer, I realized that what I was seeing was wire mesh inside the glass, designed to prevent break-ins.

In a slow drawl, he said, "Who are you—the doctah?"

"No," I said. "My name is David Farrell. I am just visiting." I stuck out my hand and said, "Nice to meet you. What's your name?"

He gave me a nice firm handshake. His hands were soft and well worn.

"Waitts. Condee Waitts," he said in a loud voice. "Who you visiting?"

"Well, the truth is, Mr. Waitts, I'm thinking about taking the job as the manager here," I responded.

Mr. Waitts grabbed my hand again. He leaned forward from his sitting position in bed, looked me straight in the eye, and said, slowly and quietly: "I think that'd be good."

At that point, I was on the fence about this whole thing. This facility looked overwhelming, and I was having serious second thoughts about taking the job. But then, BOOM! "I think that'd be good." I decided I was meant to take this on.

I never thought that I would be back to managing a nursing home so quickly; I had known I would return someday, but not now.

Being a nursing home administrator is a noble career. I heard a colleague once say that it is like being the mayor of a small town. Few jobs offer one the opportunity to positively influence hundreds of people daily and thousands annually.

I knew I wanted to be a nursing home administrator after my first encounter with one convinced me that I could do better. I was working as a nurse's aide at Braintree Manor in Braintree, Massachusetts, when I was called to the administrator's office. She gave me a written warning for being in the building while I was not "on the clock."

I explained to her that I hadn't known about the rule and that I was simply visiting with a few residents who did not seem to have very many visitors and who seemed lonely.

After my explanation, I thought she would withdraw the warning notice. But, to my shock and anger, she indicated that I must sign it and comply with the rule. I said, "You must not care about the residents." That statement clearly upset her. I signed the warning and got out of her office.

I thought a lot about the craziness of that interaction. A few weeks later, I broke the rule again to visit Grace on a Sunday. Grace was a sweet person who lived in a three-bed ward next to a sunny window, where she had a few small plants she tended. I liked talking to her. She was a good listener.

I figured I was safe since the administrator didn't work on Sunday and no one would tell the administrator that I was there. But one of the CNAs I worked with on the night shift, who was working a double that afternoon, reported me. That CNA didn't like me one bit. I am not sure why. I think she resented having to wake me up from my meal break every time we worked together.

Soon after that, I was fired—fired for visiting the residents on my own time. It was devastating. I sat in my car in the parking lot and cried, holding my termination paycheck in my hand.

That's when I decided that I wanted to manage a nursing home. I wanted to be an administrator who encouraged staff to visit with the residents. I wanted to make a difference in elders' lives.

My first experience in nursing home management came at a large facility outside San Diego. I was an administrator-in-training (AIT) under an administrator named Bob, who preached to me about the power of "the fin-ger." He told me to wave my index finger in the face of department heads when they were not performing. I'll never forget when he told me one day, "Only use the power of the finger when you really need to. If you use it too much, it loses its value."

For six long months I worked under Bob. It was torture. He insisted that I sit across from him at his large desk while he smoked cigarettes (this was 1989) and listened to country music on his radio. But what I learned from Bob was very valuable: He was the opposite of the type of leader I wanted to be.

When I was miserable and ready to quit the AIT program, my dad kept me going and encouraged me to stick with it. He came to visit us in San Diego when I was about halfway through the AIT process. When I described the terrible working conditions and how miserable I was, he replied: "You should stick it out. It is only a few more months."

At the end of the AIT program, when I was ready to go out on my own and manage a building for the large nursing home chain that employed me, I asked Bob if he had made his recommendation about me to the higher-ups and what the plans for me were. To my dismay, Bob said, "I told them that I did not think that you would be a very good administrator. I did not recommend that you take on a facility."

I could not believe it. After all that I had endured.

Thankfully, later that day, an administrator of a small facility in eastern San Diego gave her two weeks' notice, and I was given the opportunity to take over. Sure enough, I did the opposite of what Bob taught me, and the facility was quite successful. My career in nursing home administration was born.

That was 18 years ago. Since then, I have served as the administrator at several nursing homes. Along the way, in partnership with others, I estab-lished a core set of practices that continually produced positive results. It was all based on one simple but powerful theory: People respond well to being treated with trust and respect. After many years as an administrator, I worked for a few years as a quality care consultant to nursing homes through Qual-ity Improvement Organizations (QIOs). Most recently I had been at Quality Partners of Rhode Island, a support center for QIOs across the country.

I had developed my practices intuitively, by seeing what did and didn't work in the homes I was managing, so when I delved into the world of qual-ity improvement I was excited to learn that long-term care researchers had identified many of the same leadership practices as key to providing excellent care and service to nursing home residents. Now, here I was in another part of California, reentering the world of nursing home administration. I wanted to apply all I had learned and put it all together. I could test the evidence about good practice on a home whose current circumstances were producing mediocre results.

I wanted to make this home a better place to live in and work in, by implementing the principles of organizational culture change, leading it away from the institutional model toward individualized care, and taking workforce development to the next level. And I wanted to chronicle my journey, so I would have a record of the things I tried to do and the impact they had on the lives of the residents and staff. I anticipated utilizing the information to help other troubled homes and figured I may have opportunities to share what I had discovered with others in this field.

Still, walking around here for three days of orientation, I'd had my doubts. I had my doubts about my own abilities and I had my doubts about the models I was preaching. And then . . . Mr. Waitts said, "I think that'd be good."

Day 1—June 12, 2006

I felt like I was in a fog all day today. I just couldn't figure out what was what. I couldn't even figure out if all the nursing staff had shown up as scheduled. The daily staffing sheet was no help.

The pace seems frantic compared to the QIO world. My initial assessment is that there is one main person who keeps it all together here. His name is Andy, and he is the assistant director of nursing.

People here are pretty excited about the state survey results. They had by far their best inspection in years, but I've been shaking my head all day and asking how. The facility definitely does not give the impression of efficiency and organization. The environment is very shabby.

The facility received eight deficiencies but no major scope and severity issues. I was shocked because there are about nine people with pressure sores they got while they were here. In most states, that's grounds for strong enforcement action—immediate jeopardy finding, fines, a stop to new admissions, and maybe even headlines in the local paper.

This survey proves just how inconsistent survey results can be and how little stock we can place in those results unless the survey outcomes are consistent with other clinical measures and key metrics.

Day 3—June 14, 2006

I attended a regional administrators' meeting today where they announced that they have sold this small company to a larger one. An executive from the larger company presented their focus and goals. And here is how it sounded to me:

- Make lots of money.
- Don't get sued.
- Have fewer deficiencies than the state average.

- Fill beds with the highest-paying residents—Medicare. Keep them as long as possible.
- Reduce overtime and double-time.

As I listened, I was struck by how little has changed over the nearly 20 years that I have been in this profession. In fact, these are the same goals that were stated in the very first administrators' meeting I ever attended, back in 1989. Today, there was no talk of quality measures, resident quality of life, employee engagement, resident and family satisfaction, or making the shift to person-directed care.

The message was loud and clear—this is a business. The focus is the bottom line. Yet I know that the best way to a good bottom line is through good treatment of staff so that they will then provide good care. These executives know that. Why don't they express it and outline steps to get there? The presentations leaned way too heavily toward the obvious outcomes. It was missing something necessary to inspire us administrators and directors of nursing (DONs).

Now I want to make something clear. The outcome measures discussed as the goals by the executive are very important to me. In fact, I pore over the financial statements as soon as they are released. It's very important to me to exceed budgeted profitability. So, as you see, I have no problem with the goals discussed by the high-ranking executive from the new company. It's the lack of attention on other important performance metrics that bothers me.

There are simply not enough individuals in high-ranking positions in long-term care that we can look up to. It seems like the toughest rise up the ranks. At this point in my career and after having read so much of the culture change literature, I look around me at the meeting and I listen to what is being said, and I think that this is where the problem truly lies. We need more leaders who can inspire us and focus us on other performance goals.

Back at the facility, I see an environment that has been neglected by the previous administrator who was very cheap. But, historically, that's how administrators are trained and rewarded. Every line item of a profit and loss (P&L) statement is analyzed according to the measure of cost per resident per day (PPD). We calculate PPD by how much money we spend on something—say, food—and then divide it by the total number of resident days in a given month. And with the dollars PPD measure, we focus on pennies-per-day. The measure itself promotes frugality.

Day 4—June 15, 2006

I feel like I'm in a time warp. I feel like I've worked two weeks, but really I have only been here for four days.

I learned today that the housekeeping supervisor is reluctant to distribute the new linen because he does not like the CNAs hoarding the clean linen in the residents' rooms. What he doesn't know is that CNAs are survivors. If they work in a facility that does not supply enough linen to do their job, then they begin their shift by taking the linen that they can find in the linen closets and hiding it in the rooms of residents they're assigned to care for. Of course, this is a smart strategy so they have enough linen to change their assigned residents' beds and have some clean towels after giving a shower.

The housekeeping supervisor's attitude about the frontline staff here is shared by some of the department heads. They see staff as untrustworthy, lazy workers who need to be tightly managed and punished.

The staff needs the linen to take care of the residents. When I look in the linen closets throughout the halls, they are usually bare of the essentials—towels, washcloths, fitted sheets, blankets, and pillows. Treating the staff as thieves and, as a result, then not purchasing enough linen every month is crazy. It's got to stop.

End of first week—June 17, 2006

Shock and awe.

As for the staff, the late researcher from Harvard, Susan Eaton, one of my favorite long-term care researchers, was right: even those who make just $8.50 an hour do take some pride in their work and have a sense of fulfillment. However, here, the general management approach has been "enforcement" and "write people up." There's no effort to trigger that pride.

Even so, these people are survivors. I guess many of the staff have always been treated this way by their bosses, so they don't expect anything different here.

I noticed one of our restorative nursing assistants as being particularly kind and well-meaning. She's an African American woman with silver teeth who smiles all the time. She uses a loving approach with the residents that clearly lights up their day. I told her that I noticed her positive approach and attitude and thanked her for the difference she makes here. She seemed taken aback by my comments and muttered, "Really?"

"You are a positive force," I repeated.

"No one ever said that to me before," she said. "Really?"

"Just because they haven't said it does not mean it isn't so," I told her. "Thank you."

She blushed and walked away.

How could this be the first time she has heard that compliment? It's obvious how much she contributes.

This is one of the root causes of the problem. There are employees here who are living angels. They need positive feedback, and lots of it.

Day 10—June 21, 2006

I had an interesting conversation with the dietary supervisor today. I have been holding individual meetings with all of the department heads regarding their jobs, goals, and daily work schedules. She began the meeting by expressing remorse about how much over budget her food costs were. I asked what her budget was, and she said $4.75 PPD. I said, "Have you ever told someone outside of long-term care that you feed elders three meals a day for $4.75?"

She said, "No."

"I have, and they are shocked. Think about it. We cannot purchase a healthy lunch for less than $7 and we feed elders here three meals for $4.75? Amazing!"

We looked at the latest P&L statement, which revealed that the food costs were averaging $5.06 PPD. "Do the people like the food?" I asked her.

She responded, "Yes, the residents like the food."

I had been receiving a lunch tray delivered to my office daily and the food tasted good to me and presented well.

I asked, "Are the elders losing weight? What is the percentage of residents with a significant weight loss?"

"Two percent," she said proudly.

"Awesome! Then I do not really care if you are 31 cents over budget on your food costs PPD. If the residents like the food and are not losing weight then I am happy."

She had a look of shock on her face. "Wow, there's a different perspective," she said.

I have become deinstitutionalized. Fours years away from a nursing home will do that. So it feels strange for me to be back in this institutional world, facing people who have been brainwashed in the institutional ways. Clearly, she had been hammered about her food costs and expected me to do the same. A budget of $4.75 for three meals and we are spending $5.06. Wow.

Andy, our assistant director of nursing, came in next. He told me that, during the overlap between the day and evening shifts, there is a shortage of parking spaces and some nursing staff members have to double-park in the garage. When this occurs, he said, our maintenance supervisor was instructed by the previous administrator to call the city meter maids, who come to our parking lot and write tickets for the double-parked cars. Andy thought that practice was unfair.

My jaw dropped. I assured him that I would put a stop to that immediately.

I cannot believe that the previous administrator would allow such a practice. Oh wait, after seven days here, I guess I can.

I came in this morning and the night shift CNAs told me that they had had a very difficult time providing care last night because there were very few clean linens and towels to do their job. When I checked, I was amazed to find that the facility was budgeted to spend $800 a month on linen, but it had only spent $1,400 on new linen in the entire fiscal year (11 months). Some managers might see that as a good thing: The facility saved close to $9,000 on linen. But at what expense?

When towels and sheets are worn and shabby, or rough, residents' skin, which is usually fragile, is more likely to break down, creating pressure sores. This is a very painful and devastating clinical outcome.

It is also expensive. Research shows that treating one stage-three pressure sore in a flat-rate Medicaid reimbursement system costs a facility close to $9,000 to heal when you factor in dressing, ointments, and nursing staff time. When I arrived at this facility, there were six residents with in-house-acquired pressure sores.

I'm reminded of the saying, "Penny wise and pound foolish."

Day 11—June 22, 2006

Two days ago, I sat down at Nursing Station Two and something stabbed me in the back. It turns out that a very sharp object was jutting out of the back of the chair. I asked the nurse standing by her med cart, "How long has this been like this? This is dangerous."

She answered, "It has been like that for quite some time now."

I informed her that I needed to remove this chair immediately, as it was a hazard. She said, "Please don't. We are all aware of the spike in the back of the chair and we know how to avoid it."

I looked around at the other chairs at the nursing stations. They were falling apart too. I let her know I would leave it for now, but that I would take care of it. She gave me a look of doubt.

I went straight to Charlo, the central supply clerk. We ordered a couple of nice, solid office chairs for the nursing station. I let her know that I wanted her to order two new chairs a month for the next three months, until we had replaced them all.

Today, the chairs arrived and the maintenance supervisor put them together. He placed them at Station Two and removed the chair with the spike in the back and another one that was falling apart.

Later that day, I walked by Station Two and greeted the nurses sitting in their new chairs. Wow! You would have thought they had just won the lottery. The smile on their faces was just what I needed at that moment.

The lead CNA, Kiren, made my day when she pulled me aside and said, "You know, you have done more for us in two weeks than anyone has done for us in two years. The previous administrator talked about replacing the chairs at the nurses' station and talked about a lot of other things that never happened. You don't talk about it, you just do it. Thank you."

These people are not asking for a lot. They just want to sit in a chair that does not stab them in the back. My wife said to me last night, "Do not get down on what the corporate office will not let you do. Just do what you can." She was right.

Now I'm thinking, what else can I do? I'm charged up.

Day 12—June 23, 2006

I came in at midnight and was surprised to run into Andy, the ADON. He said, "Mr. David, what are you doing here?"

I am shocking Andy almost every day. The first week, he was examining my every move. This week, I have noticed that he is beginning to trust me. Certainly my being here at midnight on a Friday night helped.

I told him I was there to meet with the night shift staff and express my commitment to supporting them and getting them the supplies they need. He smiled. Andy has an infectious smile—very broad, with lots of sparkling white teeth.

Then I asked what he was doing there. He explained that this was the last shift of one of the devoted charge nurses who had worked here for the past 10 years. She was moving to Maryland to pursue an advanced degree in nursing. He said that he had brought in a cake.

I said, "Great. I ordered pizza, so this will be a nice sendoff for her."

At the meeting, after Andy's speech honoring the nurse, he turned the floor over to me. About 15 employees filled the room, representing at least eight nationalities. I asked them to line up shoulder to shoulder according to their month and day of birth. They quickly lined up, from January 14 through December 9. I then asked them to pair up and share with each other where they were born. Chatter filled the room. When the buzz died down, I asked them to share with one another the best birthday they had ever had. Again, a nice buzz filled the air.

When they were ready, I told them how proud I was of the rich diversity at our nursing home. When I mentioned that the staff speaks 19 different first languages, they clapped.

Then I explained the form they'd been asked to fill out for a new name badge. The form asks for their name, title, and place of birth. I informed them that by indicating where they were born, we honor them and celebrate the diversity we have here. In addition, adding on a name badge the place of birth helps create conversation and promote relationship building.

I turned to an Asian nurse who was working her first shift after being hired last week. I asked, "Li, where were you born?"

She said, "I was born in Seoul, South Korea."

"If you saw another employee whose name tag said Seoul, wouldn't that help to break the ice?"

She said, "Sure. I would like to see that."

The room got quiet, I lowered my voice and said, "The quality of the relationships that we have with one another determines the quality of the care our residents receive. We must be mindful that respect of one another is the foundation of healthy relationships. I care about the relationships here and will do what I can to enhance the quality of your work life here."

To my surprise, they clapped again.

End of Second Week—June 24, 2006

Despite being told that the corporation didn't allow animals in its facilities, I have brought my dog Diego to work with me since last Wednesday.

Diego grew up at a nursing home in San Rafael, California, and came to work with me there every day for over four years. That was more than four years ago, so I was amazed to see how quickly Diego adapted to our nursing home. It was like he remembered, and he seemed very happy being in that environment again. All day long, he surprised people—both the residents and the staff. After the initial surprise, he brought smiles to people's faces. He was doing his job.

On Thursday, a daughter of one of the residents came in to visit with her mother and brought her four young children with her. Their ages ranged from 3 to 11, and it was Diego that made their visit a fun one.

I showed them all of Diego's tricks—high five, roll over, crawl, chase your tail, and beg. They were having a blast, and their grandma and mom were enjoying watching them. Clearly, Diego was key in prolonging their visit, giving the elder a chance to watch her grandkids engage in an activity and creating some laughter and spontaneity. The visit was not boring for the kids because Diego was there, and next time Mom says "Let's go visit Grandma," remembering Diego will probably make them more inclined to say, "Sure, let's go."

Animals help the culture in nursing homes in so many ways. And to think I am breaking a policy by bringing him to work. It's probably only a matter of time until I get caught, but it's hard for me to follow rules that make no sense.

Day 16—June 27, 2006

The resident across the hall from me, Alice, has really taken to me and Diego.

My office is a converted resident room, so I am directly across from Alice's room. Most of the rooms are shared by two people, but there are a few three-person rooms. Alice is in one of them.

She is a petite elder with thinning, long, oily hair whose small TV is on all day long. She lives in an extremely confined space next to the doorway. This allows her to watch me go in and out of the office all day long. About eight times a day, she wheels herself over to my office and knocks on the side of the wall (my door is always open). She always says one of three things: "I am leaving at 5:00," "I am leaving at 1:00," or "Call me a cab."

I never saw her smile until she saw Diego. Now she smiles every day when she sees him. Diego, being the moocher that he is, parks right next to her in her wheelchair when he sees that her lunch tray has arrived. She loves it and gives him treats.

I know I should probably harness Diego and lock him in my office when the food trays are out, but the residents love giving him nuggets from their plates. Diego is so gentle the way he takes food from their fragile fingers. He senses their frailty.

Diego is an incredible dog. And I am not just saying that because I am a biased owner of the mutt. He really is special.

Day 18—June 29, 2006

Compared to the other meals that I have had here, today's lunch was really bad. I named it the "San Quentin Lunch." It looked bad and smelled even worse. It looked like one scoop of brown, chunky mess next to a small muffin. It was not good.

In the first 15 days of my tenure here I have focused on other areas. Right now, the kitchen overwhelms me. Once I start working on the dietary services issues I predict I will have very little time for anything else.

However, this lunch just motivated me to focus on dietary services right away. These elders deserve better than this. This is very discouraging.

Day 19—June 30, 2006

A week ago, I called a few local art schools and connected with Ruth, an art teacher who was willing to help us design and paint some murals in the interior walls of our three courtyards. She said she would charge only $200 if she could keep the leftover supplies for her art class.

Today, Ruth began painting the mural in the first courtyard. She designed an adobe-themed mural with lots of beautiful colors. It looks fantastic.

Around noon, I changed my clothes and helped paint the top of the peaked section at the highest point in the courtyard. The ladder I was using was steep and I was hanging over the inner courtyard from the second story, so I tried not to look down. I got a lot done.

The assistant activity director was helping out. Later, I saw one of the day shift CNAs, Angie, painting after her shift ended at 3:00. I walked up to her, thanked her for helping out, and told her how much it meant to me. She just smiled.

The painting was fun today. I felt so good doing something where I could see tangible evidence that I was making an impact. Being hands on and willing to do some hard, physical work is always a surefire way to gain respect from the employees. It is healthy for the organization, and it makes me feel good.

The mural looks wonderful.

The courtyards have so much potential. My vision is that the therapists and restorative aides will begin to use the patio to walk with the elders instead of just walking down the hallways. The courtyards will also be great for the residents and their families.

We are going to create an oasis here in the middle of all the chaos of our urban downtown.

Day 23—July 3, 2006

Today we had a visit from a Department of Health Services (DHS) inspector on a resident complaint. I had just gotten back from changing into a T-shirt and jeans because I was getting ready to paint. The receptionist called to tell me an inspector was here to see me. I thought she was kidding. "Are you coming out here?" she asked.

The DHS inspector did not look happy to be here. When she entered my office, Diego went to give her a greeting. "I do not like dogs," she said. I quickly took him away.

"I am here on a resident complaint regarding cleanliness of the bathrooms and poor resident care," she said sternly. "I need this resident's chart. She was discharged last week, and here is her name." She handed me a piece of paper with the resident's name on it.

She told me she was going to look at the residents' bathrooms and walked straight across the hall and into Alice's bathroom. I felt embarrassed, since I hadn't checked the bathroom in a while so I didn't know what she was going to see in there. I winced when she came out of the bathroom and made a face.

"Nasty," she said, as she walked over to the next resident's room.

I quickly checked the bathroom while Alice watched my every move. She was right—there was a pretty nasty-looking ring around the base of the toilet. It did not look good. It did not smell good.

I raced after her and asked her how the other bathroom looked. "All right," she said.

I let her know the housekeeper would clean Alice's bathroom right away, and she said, "Good."

Dealing with her was very stressful. It's like I am the enemy. Her attitude was geared toward the expectation that something was wrong here, and she was going to find it.

"As soon as I get that resident's chart I will stop looking in the bathrooms," she told me. I ran down to Medical Records to see where they were with finding that damn chart.

Andy finally appeared with it. The inspector stopped looking in the bathrooms and came back to my office.

After about an hour of examining the medical record, she said she had finished her investigation and was ready to leave. I pulled Andy aside as we were walking back to meet with her. "Please wait until she presents her entire argument before you state your case," I said. "Hear her out completely, okay?" He said he would.

She discovered that one dose of insulin had not been properly documented, and she was going to send us a deficiency. She was correct, and Andy and I accepted it. She said nothing of the residents' bathrooms.

Wow . . . It's been a long time since I last dealt with a DHS inspector, but some things never change. We are guilty until we prove our innocence.

Day 24—July 4, 2006

Today, I worked on the holiday. Came in to work wearing my jeans, painted the mural outside in the main patio, and potted some indoor plants. Painting is very rewarding. You see immediate results. Management is much more complex, and rarely do you see such immediate results.

There are a few areas in the front of the building where you can see graffiti. One area is right by the front door. It has been bothering me ever since I started here. I feel it's symbolic of the culture of mediocrity that's evident here. This morning, I decided to do something about it.

I grabbed some paint and a roller we were using for the mural and went out front and painted over the graffiti. Some CNAs followed me out and stood behind me and mocked me as I was painting the graffiti.

"Don't mess up that fancy tie of yours," said Jada as she laughed.

Patrick said, "What are you doing—real work for a change?"

"You have no clue, do you?" said Alicia. "You're not from around these parts are you? Don't you realize that we'll be tagged tonight and it will be much worse than that? You better have a lot of paint because you'll be painting again tomorrow."

I didn't care what they were saying. It felt so good. I have never painted over graffiti before in my life but I always wanted to. I always imagined that it would feel good to paint over it and I was right. It felt amazing.

You cannot underestimate how important it is for the staff to see me taking a stand against this symbol of mediocrity. I hope that I am sending a loud message that things are getting better, and I will lead the way. I think most of the hourly staff love to see their managers get their hands dirty, and I am happy to oblige.

Certainly, one of the best parts of being a nursing home administrator is the spontaneity of it. It is not a boring job. There are days like this where I can see that I am making a difference. This is fun.

Day 27—July 7, 2006

I've grown accustomed to visiting with Mr. Waitts every day. He is alert and conversational and a very nice guy.

He lives in the corner of a three-bed room. His living space is fairly small and dark even though he is next to a window, since the windows are dingy and covered with a thin wire designed to prevent break-ins. He has been complaining about his roommates a lot lately and seemed pretty down about getting the first insulin shot of his life this morning.

The room next to mine, 120, is the only private room in the whole building. A single with its own bathroom, it's a bright, cheerful room that was made even better with the completion of the mural and tree trimming outside the sliding glass door to the patio. It has a nice outdoor area with potted plants. Since I have been here, one resident was admitted and died there three days later. Other than that, it has been vacant.

On my commute here this morning, it occurred to me that we could move Mr. Waitts to room 120. It would really enhance his quality of life, and I would love to have him as my next-door neighbor. I realized that, as the administrator, I had the power to make this happen, and I knew Mr. Waitts would really appreciate this change in his living environment. This change would be so positive. I wanted that for him.

Of course, such a move goes against all nursing home business logic. After all, Mr. Waitts is a Medicaid recipient, and we could charge a private-paying resident a lot more for our one private room. But long-term care is a very unique business. Sometimes—make that most times—it's just right to go with your heart. So I decided that I would offer the room to him.

He gets around in an electric wheelchair. I walked him down and showed him the room. I asked if he would be interested in moving there. He got very quiet. When I looked at his face, I saw that he was emotionally choked up. For some reason, it hit me like a ton of bricks, and I choked up too. Finally, he managed to say, in a soft, quivering voice, "I sure would." And I could tell he could not quite believe it.

I checked in on him around 4:00 p.m., after the CNAs had moved him into his new room. He was looking at all of his clothes in his big closet. "Taking inventory," he said. Then he looked up at me from his motorized wheelchair. "Thanks very much for moving me here," he said, choking up again. I patted him on the shoulder and stepped out of his new room. As I left, I said, "Good night, Mr. Waitts."[1]

Also today, one of the CNAs, Rellicia, came to me after her annual review by the DON. She found me painting the mural on the Station Three patio. She seemed visibly upset, so I took her to my office.

When we got there she said: "The DON gave me my review and said I had an attitude problem because I have had a hard life. How dare she say I have had a hard life! I feel that is a racial comment and I don't appreciate it. It is hard working here. Maybe I have had a hard life but she shouldn't say that to me. That's not right."

I replied, "You are right, that was not an appropriate thing to say."

She went on to say, "This is the hardest I have worked for the littlest of pay. She also said a racial comment to me in the past and I complained about her. We don't get along. She has something against me. Maybe I have had a hard life."

Tears started to stream down her face. I looked around for a tissue but didn't see one, so I just sat there for a moment, feeling overwhelmed.

Then I said: "I saw your rooms and the residents you took care of and thought you did a very nice job today. Rellicia, you seem like a very competent CNA. How was the rest of your evaluation?"

"It was good," she said.

I said, "I will speak to the DON about this. I am very sorry that this occurred. Thank you for telling me about it."

Rellicia got up and left my office while wiping away her tears. I sat there dumbfounded, just rubbing my head, for about 10 minutes. I was just numb.

Day 30—July 10, 2006

Today, we had the first day where I did not hear one overhead page. It does not sound like much, after writing it down here in my journal. However, it's HUGE. What I heard when I first started here was blaring noise pollution every 10 minutes.

I heard things like, "Station Two, your lunch trays are ready," and "I need a CNA to room 209 B." It sounded awful.

On my third day here, I asked the department heads to find another way to communicate because the overhead paging was a terrible distraction for the poor residents and staff, who have to listen to it all day. Overhead paging is annoying and unnecessary, and it's part of what makes so many nursing homes feel like institutions, not homes.

It took a while to get to this day—the first without a single overhead page. After two weeks of working on it, I realized I had to immediately intervene whenever I heard one. When I heard a page, I would literally run to find the employee who used it and explain why I thought we had to stop. After a while, they would agree.

Now, finally, we have peace. The residents have peace.

The environment here seems much better than it did a month ago. People are telling me things like, "We see what you are doing. Keep it up." It is very interesting to watch how the employees react to these evidence-based changes—and nice to hear that they're happy, of course. In general, the staff here are good, decent, hard-working people. I really like them.

Day 32—July 12, 2006

Nursing homes are unusual workplaces because you're working where people live. Occasionally, as you are just walking down a hallway focused on your next task, you are stopped in your tracks by something you see or hear or both.

Today, I was taken aback as I waited for the elevator. I looked over into the day room to a group of residents who were gathered together. Someone I couldn't see was playing "When the Saints Come Marching In" on the piano.

It sounded a little rough, but then the residents started to sing along. It was touching.

Earlier in my career, I worked as an activities director. I remember being moved by the old songs the residents would sing. They seemed to know all of the words, and the lyrics were so uplifting.

We have now gone at least four straight days without an overhead page. That is some progress. It's nice and quiet, and the residents can enjoy their singing without being interrupted by an overhead page.

Day 33—July 13, 2006

I just got back from an evening meeting with the p.m. shift employees. About 20 staff members were in attendance from the dietary, nursing, and laundry departments. I kind of winged my speech, but I spoke passionately and with conviction. I said something like this:

"I'm happy to be here with you tonight for our second community meeting on the p.m. shift. I am committed to meet with you every month. The community meeting is designed to provide a forum for us to communicate. It gives me an opportunity to share with you my focus, my beliefs, and my hopes for the future here. But this is also your opportunity to tell me what you need in order to provide the residents with great care and service.

"Let's not lose sight of the fact that we care for over 105 people each night. What each of you do, each and every evening, is very important. Also, we are a very unique facility with over half of our facility devoted to caring for individuals who have had a very hard life.

"I am very proud of the staff who work here. You are an amazing group of people. Sometimes it's therapeutic to step back for a moment and reflect on the contribution we are making by providing care to people in need. Never underestimate how important your job is, or forget the difference you are making in people's lives every day here.

"It was great that we did so well with the DHS inspection, but keep in mind that there are other measures of quality that we need to pay attention to. For instance, resident and staff satisfaction, staff turnover rates, and other key measures of people's quality of life.

"We measure our quality of care by pressure ulcer rates, weight loss percentages, and the number of people who fall each month. Of course, with all three, the lower the number the better. But after four weeks on the job here, I feel we have a great opportunity to enhance the residents' quality of life as well as the quality of clinical services. There are a number of ways we can accomplish these goals. I look forward to working together to do just that.

"As you can see around you, we have already improved this room and the courtyard outside that door. But what I am talking about is far deeper than just the environment. It's about how we treat each other on a daily basis. It is very important that you get along and respect one another. Changing our name badges to reflect where we were born and hanging a map of the world by the time clock are just two ways of creating awareness that our diversity is our strength.

"My focus is improving the elders' quality of care and quality of life. How do I plan to accomplish that? By treating you very well, enhancing the relationships among the staff, and creating a nice working environment for you. I believe that the happier you are, the happier the residents will be.

"Please remember that beyond good clinical care, human beings are very responsive to your compassion and kindness. I encourage you to hold the residents' hands, rub their shoulders, give them a hug, and remind them they are loved. All people, regardless of their age, need a gentle touch and a kind word when they are lonely and confused or in pain. Good nursing is both competent and compassionate."

I wrapped up by saying in a loud voice, "Now is your opportunity to ask questions or request equipment. I am here to meet your needs. I want this to be a good place for you to work. So do not hesitate to ask me anything and I will see what I can do."

One CNA asked for another Sit to Stand machine to lift the residents, and I was so glad to be able to tell her I had already ordered it.

A dietary aide asked if the home will be unionized after the new corporation takes over. I said, "No. We are not a union facility now, and the sale of the facility does not change that."

A buzz of discussion filled the room, and then there was some laughter. Clearly, people were responding to this question about the union. Most of the staff here have second jobs in unionized nursing homes. So I added: "I don't think you need a union because you have me as your administrator. I was a nurse's aide and an activities director. I know what it's like to work in a nursing home, and I have the experience and skills to make it better for you here. I am your biggest advocate."

Silence filled the room.

After what seemed forever but was probably more like a minute, one CNA began to clap. Others joined in, until everyone in the room was clapping. That was nice.

Just then, out of the corner of my eye, I saw someone gesturing my way. It was the Domino's Pizza man with the three large pizzas I had ordered for the meeting 30 minutes earlier. Wow—what incredible timing. I ran over, paid him, and brought the pizzas back to the staff.

I said, "I got you some pizza. Thank you all for everything. Please come and see me if I can help you in any way. Thanks."

Day 34—July 14, 2006

Today I got to show a large crowd of people all of Diego's tricks. At least 25 residents were all in a circle and about 20 staff members were milling around just before a community meeting I'd scheduled for the day shift staff and the residents. I grabbed a couple of dog biscuits and went in the middle of the crowd. Diego followed close behind.

I broke off a few small pieces of the dog biscuits and started the show. Diego did all of his tricks a couple of times. We ended each one with a small piece of the biscuit and a "high five." The crowd loved it. Most of them had never seen Diego's whole repertoire of tricks. Everyone was wowed.

I had stopped bringing Diego because I was breaking a corporate directive by bringing him to work, but I've started again at the urging of the department heads and frontline staff. Clearly, they see how his spontaneity and love add life to our home. I guess I will bring him about three days per week.

The community meeting started at 2:30. It is interesting to watch people's reaction to these meetings, because they are unfamiliar with gathering as a group. It seems awkward for the staff, but they're curious so they attend.

My presentation was similar to the one I did last night, with one twist. At the end after our question and answer session, I had all the staff line up. They formed a very long line that stretched from the reception desk all the way down the hallway by the second nursing station. There must have been 45 staff members in this line.

When I got them all lined up, I simply said, "You are all outstanding people. Hopefully you feel proud of the contribution you are making to our residents' lives each day you come to work here. This is more than just a job. You are making a positive difference in people's lives. Thank you."

Then I said, "Now, turn to the person ahead of you and pat them gently on the back and tell them they are doing a great job." They did, and a great eruption of laughter and talking filled the air. It seemed to go on and on, so I let it.

After it died down a bit, I said, "Now turn around to the person behind you and pat them on the back and tell them they are doing a great job." Again, the crowd started laughing and chatting. It was great.

We're creating community by fostering the growth of healthy relationships. I was watching it play out right in front of me.

Community meetings are turning out to be a big hit here, just like they were at the other facilities I managed through the years. You really can't build community without community meetings.

Day 37—July 17, 2006

Today, I led the department heads through a root cause analysis exercise with our staff satisfaction data. A major breakthrough came when we got into a deep discussion regarding the low score on the question: Does management care about the staff?

It turns out that one of the key issues contributing to the feeling that management does not care was related to the breakdown in the system of approving, scheduling. and paying employees for their vacation time and requests for days off. These requests are initially handed to the DON, who usually approves every one. She then passes the request on to the administrator for approval, and I have been passing the form on to the payroll coordinator for payment.

Well, the staffing coordinator was being left out of the loop, so employees were being put on the schedule for times they had been approved to take off. The department heads and I could see how these errors would make the staff think we don't care about them. Time off is important to people, and we kept getting it wrong.

Thankfully, we could fix the system. We decided to test a new way of doing things:

- All employees now provide their written requests to the staffing coordinator.
- The staffing coordinator looks at the schedule and accommodates the request if possible. She then shows the request to the DON, and they discuss how it can be accommodated.
- The staffing coordinator hand-delivers the request to the administrator, who signs it.
- The staffing coordinator gives the request to the payroll coordinator, who processes it.

Clearly, fixing administrative systems are necessary to demonstrate that we care about our staff.

Day 39—July 19, 2006

I had an early-morning visit from a night shift CNA at about 7:45 a.m. Catalina explained to me that she has worked here for 20 years. In a heavy accent, she said, "I have been here through the good times and the bad. I like it here. You are doing a very good job."

I said, "Thanks. Why have you stayed here for so long?"

"I don't know," she said. "This is my home. I have been here for so long." After a long pause, she said, "There is just one thing though, Mr. David. Why is new staff paid as much as the staff who has worked here for a long time like me?"

"We do offer new employees a wage rate based on their years of experience in the field. Therefore, we may offer a CNA with five years of experience a wage that one of our current employees is earning who has five years of experience here." I went on to say, "We must offer people wages based on their experience. Otherwise, all we would have here would be new graduates, and that would not be good for resident care."

I pulled out the sheet of paper that indicated how much her wage increase was going to be. I told her, "Your rate of pay increased to $13.50 per hour. And it looks like you are one of the top paid CNAs in the entire facility. So no new hire will ever earn your hourly rate."

She smiled. It looked like she felt really good about that. She kept smiling but did not say anything. She inched her way to the door.

Finally, I said: "Thank you so much for all you have done for the residents here over the past 20 years. It's great that you have been here 20 years. Please come to see me anytime."

Day 40—July 20, 2006

Again, today, I was reminded of how administrative errors can kill organizational trust and erode the culture.

A night shift CNA waited for me this morning. Leticia is an older, African American woman with a beautiful smile, despite the fact that she needs some dental work. But the look on her face this morning told me that this was not going to be a happy visit. I had sort of expected this to happen a few times today, because it's the first payday of our new fiscal year, so all the CNAs will see the amount of their raise.

"I have a bone to pick with you," Leticia told me.

"Well, thanks for coming to see me. Please come into my office."

She stepped in and said, "I do not get why I am the only CNA on nights who didn't get a raise. I feel like I have been here for the residents. Paid my dues—you know? The amount does not even matter to me. I just want to know, why not me? Why didn't I get a raise?"

I was stunned. I thought we hadn't left anyone out. I quickly grabbed my list of CNAs and looked up her name. Sure enough, to my relief, a check mark was next to her name. "I have you right here," I told her. "You were making $11.27, and we are raising your wage to $12.00. I do not understand why that didn't show up on your paycheck. I'll look into it right away and fix it for you."

Then I added: "I am sorry."

Her facial expression immediately changed from anger to sadness. Her bottom lip started to quiver and she started to cry. I stepped from around my desk and grabbed her by the shoulders. "It was just an administrative error. It has nothing to do with you. We think the world of you. Andy has told me what a great CNA you are. I am sorry about this." I hugged her, and then I stepped back.

Leticia looked down. "I am so glad I came to see you and found out it was not me. I thought it was something I did, you know?"

Then she looked up with tears streaming down her cheeks and said, with a wide smile, "You are so nice." And she walked out of my office.

Day 48—July 28, 2006

Today, we filled all of our open nursing positions. The scheduler, Kris, said that the schedule has never had so few vacant shifts. "And the best part is, all these positions got filled with competent, caring staff. I can't believe it. These are the nicest people you are hiring!"

When I arrived here, there were eight vacant positions in the nursing department and overtime averaged about 700 hours per pay period. Today, six weeks later, we have no open positions, and we will have about 300 overtime hours this pay period. These are dramatic improvements—and all the result of just a few changes.

The first, and most significant, change was the simplest of all. I learned the second week I was here that the nursing leadership team only interviewed applicants on Tuesdays at 11:00 a.m. Plenty of applicants would come in to apply, but they were all told to return Tuesday at 11:00 a.m. Naturally, not all of them could come back and some never did.

When I learned about that, I immediately changed our policy. Now any candidates who walk in the door are given an application to fill out, and I interview them after they complete it. I told the receptionist to come find me whenever an applicant is ready. I knew that it was going to be difficult to move this place ahead until we filled all these open positions here. "Nothing I am doing is more important than meeting with a candidate for employment here," I told her.

As a result, I was able to confirm that, indeed, a lot of good candidates walked through our doors. I was also able to be more selective.

I focused on character traits, like compassion and empathy and friendliness. And I counted how often they smiled. I set candidates up to interact with residents and staff, watching them carefully to determine whether they willingly interacted with others. I turned down many candidates who clearly did not engage with others. They would not have fit in. And we hired nine new staff members, all of whom are proving to be excellent people and great employees. Some are already outperforming many of our veteran staff members, and Kris is noticing the difference.

It boggles my mind that the leadership team here could be so apathetic about hiring practices and then complain about the staffing challenges they were experiencing. They watched the staffing issues impede the care and service yet they told applicants to "come back for interviews Tuesday at 11:00 a.m." There was no sense of urgency to hire as the staff and residents suffered due to the staffing instability caused by the vacant full-time positions.

Getting a handle on the nursing staff hours is more difficult now that we are working with a full complement of staff each day. Right now, we are booking more hours than the corporation wants. But I don't want to trim people's hours. Our occupancy rate will go up, and when it does our hours PPD will be right where it needs to be. Meanwhile, I will be patient and leave the nursing hours where they are as we prepare to be successful.

It is an incredible challenge to try to stay within the budget and manage the nursing hours, primarily because the denominator—the number of residents in the house—can only be predicted. Trying to adjust hours daily to fit a changing census can be a nightmare.

My philosophy is that the key is to focus on the total number of nursing hours per day, not the hours PPD. Focusing on actual hours lets the staff feel secure, knowing they can rely on a consistent, steady schedule. Good staff will leave a facility if their hours are cut every time the census dips, so I set a target of total number of nursing hours each day and aim for it. This keeps it simple for the staffing coordinator and the nursing leaders here. As we have started to consistently hit that targeted total nursing hours these past few weeks I have started to feel a positive change occurring.

Here are some specific outcomes we have accomplished in the past six weeks:

- Filled all eight of our vacant nursing staff positions
- Reduced overtime and double time from 1,400 hours a month to 600 hours
- Reduced call-offs in the nursing department from 58 in April to 23 in June.

How did that happen? I think we have made some positive changes, such as the following:

- Started interviewing everyone who walks in and applies for a job instead of telling them to come back on Tuesday at 11:00. That increased the number of viable candidates, allowing us to be more selective and choose better candidates.
- Offered an employee referral bonus to staff for referring their friends to work here.
- Made good selections, hiring people who are performing very well.
- Enhanced the environment, making it prettier, cleaner, and quieter.
- Started community meetings to bring people together.
- Started HR meetings to focus on our staff and the schedules.
- Started Employee and Rookie of the Month programs to recognize our top performers.

I think the new staff are also responsible for the drop in call-offs. For one thing, filling all of the vacant positions meant that fewer shifts are consistently left open and available for anybody to pick up. So now, a staff member can't call off sick and then easily pick up a shift later in the week. It's becoming apparent to staff that you should come to work as scheduled. All of this is leading to less and less overtime each day.

It's interesting how it's all so interconnected. Just a couple of key changes and a few new good new employees can lead to some very good business results. I'm very happy to see this. Business results like these will allow me to continue with the culture change journey here.

Day 30—July 31, 2006

I had an interesting discussion with the assistant administrator today.

Last week, when I attended a conference, I called, and she informed me that she was suspending three employees for attendance issues. I asked her to wait until we had a chance to discuss it, but she said it was already done. I let her know that I was shocked and disappointed.

As I drove home, I started thinking about how it made no sense to suspend an employee due to attendance issues. What message are we sending to this person? "You are so important to our organization that when you call off it causes great hardship. As punishment for not coming to work, we forbid you to come to work for three days." That makes no sense at all to me.

But the assistant administrator believes in the power of punishment. She has only one tool in her toolbox—a hammer. When I got back, I began our talk by asking, "Why, all of a sudden, would we suspend three employees all on the same day? Did you randomly just pick a day to review attendance records and decide to punish three worst offenders?"

She got defensive. "These employees make it hard on everyone else when they call off," she said. "It is a tremendous inconvenience. In the past, when we have suspended people for three days their attendance has improved."

"I have a hard time believing that," I told her. "Perhaps, in a few rare cases where the employee is intentionally and willfully calling off, it may be effective. However, based on my experience and the research regarding absenteeism, punishment does not address the root cause of why an employee is continuously calling off. That root cause is complex. Punishment is simple. Complex problems require complex, multifaceted solutions."

Returning to the employees' attendance records, I asked: "Did you intervene after every call off? Did we ask the employees what was keeping them from coming to work as scheduled? Did we refer them to the Employee Assistance Program? What makes you think that a three-day suspension will solve their absenteeism problems?"

"The punishment works because you hit them where it counts—their pocketbook," she said.

Reliving this tonight as I write it down, I realize that I got pretty pissed off at her reply. I said, "These are CNAs making less than $12 an hour. They are the working poor. Losing three days of pay hurts them a lot. I am not in favor of that type of punishment of people working here. And I will not allow it."

To which she responded, "It is the corporate policy. I am following the policy. Suspension is the next step in the progressive discipline process."

I said, "We will not blindly follow corporate policies that hurt people and their families and make no sense. I am not a trained seal. I will make decisions here based on what is sensible and in the best interest of the organization and the individual staff member, always giving them the benefit of the doubt."

She just shrugged her shoulders. Her facial expression showed me that she did not agree. I am losing interest in working beside her.

Day 51—July 31, 2006

Empowerment and involvement don't come easily. The staff is not jumping at the opportunities presented to them. They do not seem very motivated to participate.

Today we scheduled a general staff meeting to review the staff satisfaction survey results. I followed the advice I have been providing to nursing home leaders around the country:

- Measure satisfaction
- Post the results for staff to review
- Hold meetings with the staff regarding the results
- Use root cause analysis tools in the meeting to drill down into why certain questions scored so low.

Well, I waited and waited and not one staff person came to the meeting. The general staff notices were posted all over the building. Why? Doesn't anybody care?

There is a sense of apathy here. There is a culture of mediocrity. This nursing home and the people who work here have been neglected for so long that my six weeks of effort to make change has not broken the current culture. And why would I think that I could?

Sometimes I think we are making great strides. Other days, the barriers feel overwhelming. Cultures are strong, whether they are good or bad. I guess that's what makes them cultures. This one is strong, and the personalities here are too.

I need to find another way to get at the truth behind the satisfaction survey results. Maybe I'll just start interviewing the staff. Or I could invite a few to join me in my office to talk about it.

It sure was easier to present this stuff at a conference than it is to actually do it. I am wiped out and discouraged . . . nobody cares.

Day 53—August 2, 2006

Our in-house acquired pressure ulcers spiked up to over 6%. So today, I called a quality improvement meeting right after the morning meeting with the department heads.

I came armed with a few slides we used at the QIO. The bullet points on the slides asked questions designed to provoke a discussion that would help nursing home managers identify the gaps in their pressure ulcer prevention process.

I began the meeting by explaining how we were going to examine the system. As soon as I finished, the DON said: "I just need to write up all the nurses. This is not acceptable."

I said, "You think that's the solution? No, absolutely not. You are not to punish the nurses. If solving this complex problem was as simple as handing out written warnings, we wouldn't have a problem."

She looked dumbfounded. She really needs to go away so I can replace her with Andy, the ADON. I know that sounds harsh, but it's reality. She is not a leader. I have to make this change.

Day 54—August 3, 2006

Something interesting happened today.

We hired a gang member.

I knew this was a very bad hire the moment I came back from a meeting and I saw someone I had not seen before vacuuming the living room. I quickly learned that the housekeeping director had hired someone without my input and it turns out that he hired a gang member.

Shortly after I had sat down at my desk, two CNAs came into my office and informed me of the bad hire. They said that this guy was dangerous and was up to something. I had heard that gang members try to get into nursing homes to steal narcotics. "Do you think that's why he's here?" I asked.

"Maybe, I don't know," said Cassie, a day shift CNA. "We're just trying to give you a heads up, Mr. David, that you've been trying so hard to make this place better and that this guy that got hired . . . he's bad news, Mr. David. He's bad news."

As soon as I found out he'd been hired, I pulled the housekeeping director into my office and said, "This guy is not your answer to the vacant position you have. I want you to pretend that you didn't fill the position. That's how aggressively I want you to start looking for someone else. This guy is going to quit without notice, and he will be nothing but trouble for you while he is here. You need to watch him. We all do."

Sure enough, my predictions came true. He was loud and disruptive. He was distracting the CNAs from doing their work while standing in the hallways pretending to be pushing a vacuum. He seemed to be scoping out the medication rooms.

His behavior escalated on payday last Friday after a mistake on his check meant he would have to wait until the following payday to get paid. That led to the incident with the maintenance director, where they almost came to blows. We had a reason to terminate him and we quickly did.

I told the maintenance director I would give the man his final paycheck when he came to collect it. The receptionist alerted me when he arrived and I met him in the front of the building, in front of a bank of huge windows. Though I didn't know it at the time, all of the employees and the residents in the lobby and dining room were watching my interactions with him through these windows. They knew this guy was a threat. And clearly, this was the highlight on the activities calendar that day.

Things started out fine but quickly turned sour when he said there was another mistake on the check I had just handed him. He said, "Let me give you a heads up. I am pressing charges against Dan for pushing me two days ago. I've already got a lawyer, I know where he lives, and you are going to get called to the witness stand. What are you going to say? So, I am just letting you know that you'll be hearing from my lawyer."

All the while as he saying this, he was circling me. He was wearing big, dark sunglasses so I couldn't see his eyes. His baseball cap was on sideways. He was posturing like he was ready to slug me. I started to think about the start date of my dental insurance.

I said, "Okay. Your lawyer will talk to our lawyers. Thanks for the heads up." We went back and forth about this lawsuit thing for about five minutes as he continued to circle me while raising his voice at times. Finally, out of nowhere, a car sped up and screeched to a halt right in front of the building. The driver screamed, "Get in! Now!" He jumped into the car and they sped off.

When I walked back in, I saw Pam, one of the day shift CNAs, at the front door. As I passed by her she mumbled something under her breath.

I said, "What was that, Pam?"

"I got your back," she said.

I was touched. She had my back? Really? Wow, I thought. The culture in this home has come a long way. She had my back!

Now . . . I wouldn't mess with Pam. Pam is a strong African American woman from the city. She's tough. She knows she's tough. She smokes cigars.

"Thanks," I said to Pam. "That's so nice. You had my back."

"This is the city," she said. "But don't worry, I got your back."

Day 58—August 7, 2006

It's never a good thing when you walk into the nursing home you're in charge of and the first thing you see is the licensed nurses with concerned looks on their faces huddled around the staffing book at 7:45 a.m. That's a sure sign of a problem, which will result in a lot of shuffling around of the staff. What's even more troubling is when the shuffling starts after the start of a shift, after staff have already started their routine. Either way, you can expect some drama to play out when the charge nurses gather the CNAs to distribute the residents and the tasks of the employees who did not show up as scheduled.

It's often the nice, understanding, restorative aides who save the day by agreeing to provide direct care to a group of residents. We routinely pull them to provide that care, and so do thousands of other nursing homes. It solves the temporary staffing shortage—but it can result in some serious long-term consequences for the residents. Restorative aides keep the elders moving. When they are pulled off of their duties in order to take a CNA assignment, the elders usually do not get to move.

We have our staffing challenges, just like other facilities. I'm beginning to realize that I need to do a lot of education for our staffing coordinator, Kris. Granted, that's a really hard job. She is the most harassed person in the building. She's a good person, and I am confident that my investment in her knowledge base and capacity will pay off.

I uncovered the following while Kris was gone for a few days:

- The master monthly schedule had not been updated to clearly indicate additions, deletions, and other key changes.
- There were errors made when transferring information from the master monthly schedule to the daily master schedule.
- Staff were not filling out the required forms to ask for days off.
- Licensed staff were not filling out call-off forms when CNAs called off to work.
- The staff phone number list was not kept up to date and was not accessible to licensed nurses and managers who were attempting to fill vacant shifts.

As a result, chaos ensued.

We seem to be making a lot of administrative errors here—first payroll and now scheduling. No wonder the frontline staff does not seem to trust me or the managers. But we can correct this. We can do better than this. We need to get organized.

I took the lead and organized a new master monthly schedule book.

- I threw away the old book and replaced it with a new notebook.
- I inserted the following tabs: notes, monthly schedule CNAs, monthly schedule licensed staff, daily staffing sheet.
- I clearly indicated on the top of each schedule: shift, discipline, location, month, and year.
- I changed paper colors to differentiate between licensed staff schedules and CNA schedules.
- I put the updated staff phone number list in the book.
- I created new forms: Trading Shifts, Request for Time Off, and Call-Off.

The schedules change daily, and Kris has to keep the master monthly schedules up to date with every change. It means changing them four, five, six times a month, which includes replacing the old schedules in the staffing books and distributing the new, updated schedules to key staff. It's a lot of work. But these subtle changes lead to efficiencies for the staff by making it easier for everyone to quickly find the staffing information that they need.

I feel like I have a good handle on this now. Tomorrow I will share my ideas about addressing absenteeism at our weekly HR meeting.

Day 59—August 8, 2006

This morning, the assistant administrator, Liz, handed me the newspaper and said, "This is one of the worst stories I have seen about nursing homes." The headline read, "Nursing Homes Receive Poor Grades."

The story described a report released by an advocacy group that ranked nursing home care based on DHS inspection results. It then listed the nursing homes in our area that had made the list of the worst facilities, calling them "the ones to avoid."

One of the homes on the list was there because of poor survey results from 2000 to 2003. In the world of long-term care, that's a lifetime ago. Nursing homes are such fragile ecosystems that the quality of care and service can change in a week. To judge a facility today based on DHS inspection results from three years ago is absurd.

Sure enough, the current administrator was quoted in the paper as saying, "Those results were long ago under different ownership. We have invested in staffing and the building and our recent survey results are fine."

I said to Liz, "This could be you or me quoted in here. The results here, at this home, were just as bad from 2000 to 2003. This is ridiculous. To make claims regarding the quality of current care with data that old. In addition, it's data from one source—DHS inspection results."

Day 60—August 9, 2006

I have come to notice that there is only one meeting each month where all the important people from the corporate office get on the line to talk about your nursing home. The topic of that meeting is the facility's monthly financial performance—profit and loss. Only the P&L meeting brings the important people together.

We do so much more than just make and spend money. Why don't we have an important conference call every month regarding the quality indicators or fall prevention or reducing turnover? Why is it that we only meet with urgency when the topic is our financial performance? Don't they see that if we paid attention to the other areas, the process measures, the financial performance would improve?

This time around, I was called on to explain why my nursing hours and food costs were over budget. I became frustrated because I felt no one on the call was acknowledging that we exceeded budgeted profitability by over $70,000 and had a profit margin of over 14% (which is very good for a nursing home). Not one of the executives on the call acknowledged that we had far exceeded anyone's expectations regarding profit. Instead, they focused on a few places where we spent more than expected.

My explanation of the food costs went over like a ton of bricks. I said, "Our food is still pretty marginal. It has improved some. However, the thought of trying to cut food costs seems foolish if the food is still lacking in quality. Maybe what we are spending should be the budget. Clearly, $4.75 per resident per day for all three meals is not enough." I heard heavy sighs of disgust from the vice president of finance.

They didn't like my explanation of our nursing hours any better. I said, "I do not think we are over budget. I think the nursing hours budget is too low. I believe the 451 hours we are staffing each day is just right to provide good care here."

Again, that was met with heavy sighs and snide remarks.

After the P&L call, my boss called me. She was probably sensing my despair. While I had her attention, I presented the need to keep the resident-to-CNA ratio low.

She wanted me to cut CNA hours on the evening shift so we could get our nursing hours in line with the corporate budget. I presented the following arguments for keeping them higher:

- It is dangerous to increase the resident-to-CNA ratios at 3 p.m. Resident care and service needs do not drop off at 3:00, so there is no justification for the decrease in hours from a work-flow perspective. On the contrary, evenings are very busy. From 3 to 8 p.m. we have many visitors, new admissions, a meal to serve, residents to engage with, and others to assist to bed. Staffing at a ratio of 11-to-1 results in the CNAs starting to put their residents to bed as soon as they come on duty so they can get to them all in time, and that diminishes individualized care and quality of life for the residents.
- Evening shift CNAs come from working day shifts someplace else. They are tired when they arrive and not so quick on their feet.
- Having one extra CNA for the evening shift is an investment of just $43,000 per year, including the cost of benefits. It is a small investment with big returns.

I have been through the budget process many times, and I know there's a lot of guessing involved in creating one. So here we are beating our projected profitability by a large margin while coming in over budget in nursing hours and food costs. If we were in line with budgeted labor hours and food costs, would we have made more money?

Maybe spending a little more on nursing hours and food actually resulted in the higher profitability. Maybe what we are doing is a better formula than the budget created last year. Our results certainly indicate that.

Day 68—August 17, 2006

Earlier this evening, I led the community meeting for the evening shift. I introduced our facility mission statement and our four core values—respect, responsibility, caring, and compassion. I then introduced 19 Hospitality House Rules (HHRs).

The HHRs are a good way to introduce person-directed care and the concept of hospitality in long-term care. I have been using them ever since I saw a similar concept hanging behind a nursing station at Kaiser Hospital in Santa Rosa in the early 1990s. I adapted that list for long-term care and added many new ones. It is always better to spell out the behaviors and actions that you expect of people rather than to use vague generalities.

I explained to the staff that consistently practicing these behaviors will allow us to demonstrate our values, so we can achieve our mission.

I noticed that several of our residents were listening as intently as any staff member. After the meeting had ended, a new resident named Glenda called me over. "Oh my gosh," she said, "that is exactly what we want! That was excellent. Everything you said was true. You really hit the mark there."

I had never seen her so excited.

"I used to work the graveyard shift, so my body clock is backwards," she went on. "I want to stay up late at night. So what you said about honoring our requests and treating us as individuals is true. Thank you so much."

Mr. Waitts was there as well. "That was a nice speech." he said in his slow drawl. "You sure are good." He grinned and nodded slowly.

That made me feel really good.

Day 69—August 18, 2006

I made a couple of tough personnel decisions this week. I informed the company that we contract with for housekeeping, laundry, and maintenance services that they needed to find me another supervisor. I also informed the accounts payable clerk that she was not cutting it and would be moving back to her old job as admissions assistant.

Telling people the hard truth about their performance is never easy. In the past, I might have put these tough conversations off, but not now. I don't like to make anyone feel sad, but to move this organization forward, I must have these difficult conversations.

After investing a considerable amount of time over the last couple of months in coaching the housekeeping supervisor, I had to tell him today: "You're just not taking my feedback seriously enough. I have been very specific about my expectations of you. Unfortunately, you are consistently not meeting those expectations. It is a combination of lack of effort, poor judgment, and simply not taking responsibility."

He just shrugged.

The more experience I get as a leader, the more convinced I become that you should give people honest feedback on their performance when their performance isn't up to your expectations. Do it in a kind way, but do it right away. Don't delay. And be straightforward so there's no doubt about what is being said.

Day 72—August 21, 2006

I don't like Mondays anymore. I bet most nursing home administrators feel the same way. Mondays stink.

I used to *love* Mondays in the QIO world, since they're usually pretty quiet. But, as I have learned over the past eight weeks, they're not so quiet when you are a nursing home administrator.

I think it has something to do with the fact that there isn't any time on a Monday morning to settle in, shake off the weekend, and get into work mode. Right off, you're hit with what happened over the weekend, and it's rarely good news, at least not in a facility you're trying to turn around.

So many things can go wrong over the weekend. This past weekend, a whole boatload of staff called off from work. Someone fell and was sent to the emergency room. A family member complained that Saturday's lunch was horrible. The night shift ran out of Attends and was using sheets and towels as adult briefs instead. And on and on and on. . . .

I really don't like Mondays anymore.

Day 82—August 31, 2006

Today, I experienced the tears of three employees.

At 9:00 a.m. I was summoned to the downstairs business office because Diane, one of our CNAs, was crying. Apparently she injured her arm moving a resident, and she seemed to be in severe pain. I immediately referred her to our clinic, sending her on her way when she said she could drive.

A white Anglo-Saxon woman, slight of build and with decaying teeth, Diane had been doing well, I thought. I had checked in with her constantly during her first two weeks, as I do with all newly hired staff, and she seemed content.

But Kris, the staffing coordinator, pulled me aside after Diane left for the clinic. "I think that girl is on meth," she said.

"What makes you say that?" I asked.

"Well, through my church I help people who are on drugs, and she looks like them."

"Are you sure? She was doing very well." I was hoping she wasn't sure. After all, I hired Diane. But Kris said she had changed over the past few days. "I am pretty sure she's using drugs."

I went back to my office and stared at nothing until I had a thought. I called the assistant administrator and told her to give Diane the number of the Employee Assistance Program (EAP) we have a contract with. She said she would do it.

Shortly after returning to my office, I was called down to meet with another employee who was crying in the assistant administrator's office. This time it was the unit supervisor, Elli. She was pretty hysterical.

"They don't help me," she sobbed in a heavy Russian accent.

"Who?" I said.

"The nurses!" She screamed. "They don't measure the wounds when I need them. And Natasha, she's on the phone for eight hours. She never gets off the phone. They won't even write the resident's name on the bottom of a new page for the chart. I have to do it. I have to do everything. Nobody helps me." Basically, though she didn't realize it, she was saying: "I am not an effective supervisor."

"Elli, it sounds like people are not responding to your approach," I said. "What are you going to do differently?"

She was speechless for a moment. Then she said, "I guess I will write them all up."

"NOOOOOOOOOOOOooooooooooo! That is not an effective approach. Elli, maybe we are not playing to your strengths in this role. What is your favorite part of the job?"

"I don't have one. I want to spend time with the residents more. I am doing so much paperwork."

"So, a charge nurse position may be good for you. That way you can do what you do best. We want you to be happy and successful here, Elli. Would you consider changing positions?"

"Sure."

The third person who cried was the DON. She was let go today.

The corporate executives had been talking about asking for her resignation for a long time now. I admit, I prompted the action by pursuing it with my boss. Again, this was a tough personnel decision, but the right one to move the organization along to the next level in service and care.

These things are never easy. It is so easy to do nothing instead of dealing with it. No one likes to upset people. Especially me.

In his book *Good to Great*, Jim Collins writes: "People are not your most important asset—the right people are." Those words really resonate for me now. Repeating that quote helps me to cope with the discomfort of causing another person emotional pain.

So, three people cried today. Not me though. I didn't cry today. That was last week.

Day 87—September 5, 2006

Some days are just a blur, but at the end of the day, a few things linger in my mind. Like the sight of a resident dying.

It's hard. I have not had to experience this in awhile.

Ms. Gonzalez called me into room 215 while I was saying "hello" during my morning rounds. I looked at her roommate and saw that she was dying. She was really gasping for air into the oxygen mask. A large oxygen tank sat beside her. She was struggling to live. She was thin as a rail and her thin skin seemed taut against her sharp cheek bones.

Her daughter was there, as she had been so many times before.

"Can I get you or your Mom anything?" I asked.

"No."

This is the part of the job I didn't miss when I worked for the QIO. The deaths.

Human beings die in nursing homes. Employees here face more death in a year than most people do outside of this environment in their entire lifetime. I am taken aback by it now. I was used to it before.

Few jobs have this element of death. In the safe haven of the cubicle world I occupied for the past four years, there was virtually no chance that I would stumble upon a human dying in the next cubicle. But here, in this "abnormal" work environment, death can be around any corner, in any room.

Sometimes I think it's a good thing I have not become immune to death. When I become immune, I think, that's when I'll know I should get out of the profession for good.

Other times, just the opposite thoughts swirl in my head.

Here I was this morning cruising through my rounds, focused on the organization, thinking about those 10 things on my "to-do" list. Preparing for the next quality improvement meeting. After all, I am running this business. And then, just like that—WHAM! Here's a slap of reality. Look here. A human being is dying right in front of me. Right there. She's dying.

I'm human. This is rough. And this is the only thought that stuck with me from today as I sit down to write this tonight.

Day 88—September 6, 2006

People really appreciate just being asked. Just today I asked Letu, one of the evening shift CNAs, "Is everything going well for you here? Is there anything I can do to make it better for you? Do you have enough linen and supplies to do your job? Do you have plenty of lifts?"

Letu is a quiet, steady worker. She shows up every day on time and with a smile on her face. She treats the residents with respect. I notice how consistently good she is, and I want to keep her here. I want her to be happy, so I'm interested in what she has to say.

She didn't have a request for me, but the smile she gave me as she said she was fine let me know that she liked being asked these types of questions.

All the leadership gurus write that workers need to be asked how they're doing, but I don't think many managers actually take time to do it. Yet it's so powerful, even therapeutic, for staff members to know the boss cares enough to ask the right questions. The breakthrough for me is that it's these questions that state—I care about you and the residents!

Of course, being genuinely interested in the answers and willing to act on them counts for a lot too. But I don't have to know all the answers. I just have to remember the right questions to ask.

We have made some significant progress over these past three months:

- Overhead paging has been completely eliminated.
- All the vacant positions in the nursing department are filled, and we've started a waiting list for CNAs who want to work here.
- Monthly staff call-outs have declined by 50% since June.
- The nursing staff does not work short staffed anymore.
- We have established a new leadership team.
- Physically, the building has never looked better.
- The staff seems happier.
- Occupancy has gone way up.

I am feeling pretty good about our progress, but many challenges lie ahead. I'm still working at what Jim Collins calls "getting the right people on the bus, the wrong people off, and the right people in the right seats." We're "turning that giant heavy flywheel" in the right direction. But the residents still look bored and sad.

A lot of staff members have made positive comments to me lately. That's really keeping me going right now because I feel as if I've hit a wall. I got a real boost when Mia, a CNA who has been here for the past three years, stopped me in front of my office today and said, "Everything you have done here is just great. All the new colors are beautiful. Thank you."

Mr. Waitts was right there, and he heard what she said. After she walked away I looked over at him and he gave this very warm, approving, grandfatherly smile. It's nice having him as a neighbor.

Day 90—September 8, 2006

All the staff appeared very open to renaming the nursing stations from Stations One, Two, Three, and Four to our city neighborhood names. I proposed this to give our home more of a community feeling. I expected more people to question the intent, but that didn't happen. I was a little surprised. I expected more jaded, sarcastic comments. I noticed their absence and felt great about it.

This afternoon, I went to each nursing station and spoke to small groups of the nurses and CNAs. I told them what we were doing and why and asked which name they preferred.

Clearly, they liked the concept. They especially liked being asked what name they'd like for their neighborhood. The one they work in every day.

These name changes may seem like a small, quirky, culture change artifact. But someday when I look back on this, I think it will prove to have been a significant change because it opens the door to many other significant changes, such as these:

- Neighborhood CNA peer mentors
- Neighborhood meetings
- Neighborhood-specific quality data
- The concept of four distinct neighborhoods within a community.

In trying to move from institutional to individualized care, I find, some changes are easy to make while other changes are met with tremendous staff resistance. It's hard to predict what changes will come easily in a nursing home. One thing is certain and I'm realizing this as we go here—there's no need to overanalyze it. Just change something for the better. And then change something else. Keep pushing the "flywheel" in the same direction—toward person-centered care. That's what I'm doing and that's what I'm going to keep doing.

Jim Collins's findings in *Good to Great* sure resonate with me today. His research team found that it's the culmination of many little changes, not one or two big changes, that transforms organizations from good to great.

Every Friday afternoon, I get this urge to do something, anything, to beautify our community just a little bit more. Environmentally, the building is starting to look better and homier each week.

Today, in my Friday afternoon effort to make the place look just a little nicer, I planted flowers in two square blue pots and placed them on either side of our front door. I had been eying these two blue pots at Home Depot for awhile, just knowing they would look great out in the front of the entrance here. Last week, when I saw them on sale and knew we could afford them, I finally bought them, and I was right—they look great.

Day 93—September 11, 2006

Back to who's on the bus and who's gotten off the bus. So far this month, we've made three key personnel changes that will significantly help this organization implement person-directed care. The DON was asked to resign, the assistant administrator resigned, and today we asked for the resignation of Rita, who was, in my opinion, our worst-performing CNA.

From the very first day I arrived, I saw Rita display body language and facial expressions that made me cringe and put frowns on the faces of the residents. Her personnel file was littered with warnings for everything from swearing when she was at the nursing station to excessive tardiness to verbal altercations.

I realize some may say that we should "coach them, work with them, don't give up on them." And I have definitely tried that approach with many individuals through the years. But when it doesn't work and residents' comfort and security, maybe even their lives, and at least their quality of life, are at stake, well . . . then . . . changes have to be made.

Trying to coach someone who is not there for the right reasons, displaying little if any empathy or affection and respect for the residents, leaves everyone vulnerable. The residents are suffering right now, and the longer you keep this person around, the more they will suffer. Staff suffers too, because they're working right alongside someone who's having a negative impact. And the high-performing staff are looking for us, the leaders, to take responsibility and make sure they have good co-workers alongside them.

If the quality of long-term care is all about relationships, then it's also all about quality people who have the capacity to form close relationships with others. We will never become "great" until we replace our marginal and poor performers, not just with better workers, but with better human beings.

I guess I have been writing a lot lately about personnel changes. That's because I'm experiencing what feels like a bit of a breakthrough: I'm learning that creating positive outcomes in long-term care facilities is more complicated than just creating excellent systems. You have to have great communication among the human beings working in the systems. And great communication is dependent on their positive relationships.

A group of people with strained relationships will break the most perfectly designed system.

Day 94—September 12, 2006

People seem to be responding very positively to the new colors being used to paint some of the common rooms around the facility. It is truly amazing what some paint will do to an old, institutional facility. Maharaj, our full-time painter (beautification specialist), has been here for two months, and he has done a world of good.

I was able to fit Maharaj into the budget by coding his hours to the dietary department as a dietary aide. We had plenty of hours in the dietary budget, and sometimes you just need to be creative with your budgeted labor hours. It's always been my experience that the most effective administrators simply find a way to be successful under the constraints of any budget.

Many of the paint colors we are using here I used for my own home. Maharaj used the Chestnut Red my wife and I chose for our home in one of the neighborhood dining rooms—and wow! What a drastic change from the institutional green and gray colors that were everywhere in the facility three months ago. The home is just much more visually appealing than it has ever been.

It's difficult to determine the response from the residents. But for the staff, it's been a completely different story. They openly express their appreciation for the new colors. And I think they like the effort being made to beautify the place.

"I love the red," said Carl, the restorative aide, with a wide grin.

"The blue and yellow look so good together. How did you choose those two colors?" asked Lila, the charge nurse.

"My wife chooses them," I responded. "She really picks some nice colors, doesn't she?"

One thing is certain, if the staff likes it, then it has a positive spillover effect—any positive change that puts the staff in a good mood is good for the residents as well.

Day 95—September 13, 2006

Measures, measures, and more measures.

There aren't many professions where your performance is measured in as many ways as a nursing home administrator's. Daily, we administrators are judged by occupancy rates, the mix of the residents in the beds, overtime, nursing hours. Weekly, there are even more measures: workers' comp claims, collection of money owed, percentage of residents with pressure ulcers, part B revenue. . . . Finally, there are monthly measures, like the P&L statement, occupancy rates again, collections, and on and on it goes. . . .

It's hard to get all those numbers to look good all the time. There are always a few that do not look so hot. I believe corporate executives miss the point when they focus on a few numbers that are off rather than the big picture. The truth is, some numbers are just more important than others.

For example, during the last P&L call regarding August results, I found it odd that my boss pointed out that the activities department spent 49 cents per resident per day when the budget was 29 cents. The total variance was $300.

I wanted to shout, "Who cares?"

We exceeded our budgeted profit margin by over $85,000. Our profit margin was 19%, in an industry that averages 2 to 4%.

No one mentioned that the management fee of $110,000 in August was way over budget. I don't care about the management fee. It's their money and they can do what they want with it. My point is that the P&L call should have been over in two minutes. Everyone should have been happy with the big number on the bottom line. And maybe spending more on activities for the residents had something to do with that.

Unfortunately, it was not over in two minutes. For the second month in a row, I hung up with a sour taste in my mouth. I felt angry and frustrated. I took a walk around the block to cool off instead of doing rounds.

I still find it odd that the P&L call is the only really important meeting we have with the corporate staff each month. Regarding resident care and all the measures that come with it, if your facility is not due for its annual inspection by DHS, it seems that those numbers are just not that important to the corporate staff because we don't have important meetings to discuss them. The finances are a completely different story—those numbers always matter. But the key process measures—resident and family satisfaction, staff morale, quality improvement, physician satisfaction, pharmacy consultant reports, and the others . . . well—no meetings are held.

Day 102—September 20, 2006

As soon as I saw the subject line on the email from my boss, my heart sank. It simply said, "Dog."

I put off opening the email. I knew what it was going to say. I had planned to treat myself to a good breakfast at a cool place on Grand Avenue, and I knew it would ruin my mood if I read it.

But I felt compelled to read it, so I opened it. It read:

> David,
> I received an anonymous call from someone who said that they see your dog in the facility. I know that we had discussed this and I indicated that the dog was not allowed. Has the dog been going to work with you?
> Sam

What a bummer.

I knew who had told him about the dog. It was the nurse consultant who was here yesterday.

I called my boss. He cited the following reasons why the dog is not allowed:

- The liability insurance company will not allow it. It is a risk to have a dog because of biting.
- The state surveyors will cite you for infection control violations.
- If I let you do it, then I have to let others do it.

He would not even allow me to express my reasons for bringing Diego. Clearly, he was not interested in a discussion.

How insane. I ask myself, "It is 2006, right?" Having dogs and cats in nursing homes is a basic principle of culture change. It has been around since I was a nurse's aide back in the mid-1980s.

I feel angry, sad, and mad. But I know what I will do. I will gather all the evidence that counters his reasons and present it to him when the new company takes over. There is no way that the new company could have a policy against dogs.

I will speak to our liability insurance carrier and the DHS. In addition, I will gather a boatload of research that shows how having dogs in nursing homes benefits residents and staff. He can't ignore all the evidence against his decision. Can he?

But meanwhile, I have to stop taking Diego to work. I feel terrible about it, but I have to do as I was directly asked to do. I feel really mad about this. I feel really bad about this. People love that dog. He was part of the equation; he was one of the variables that is positively affecting the organization.

I keep asking myself, "This is 2006, right? Is this really happening?"

This is not good.[2]

Day 103—September 21, 2006

Andy, now the DON, came to see me today to say that he was concerned about what people will say because we have been hiring so many people from Nigeria and other African countries. He was afraid he'd be accused of favoritism, because he is from Nigeria himself. "About eight months ago, someone made a comment to that regard," he said. "I do not want to be accused of that."

I responded, "Andy, since the moment I arrived, I made it a policy that I will conduct the initial screening of applicants for all departments. It just so happens that the people from Nigeria and Ghana and other countries in Africa consistently pass my screening. I am screening for the character traits of excellent caregivers—empathy, compassion, friendliness, and a warm smile. The applicants we've had from Africa possess those traits and have been good people to hire.

"It's not really a coincidence that you are from Nigeria either. Let's face it, health care workers from Africa are applying because of you. However, you would not even interview them if they did not pass my screen. So I don't think anyone can accuse you of favoritism."

One of my foundational screening tests is the five smile rule. I don't hire people who do not smile at least five times during my initial interview. After all, people who don't smile in the interview will most certainly not smile after you hire them.

People who willingly and consistently smile at other people have a much easier time forming and sustaining warm relations with others. Caregivers who smile at the elders are the type of people I want working for us.

Day 108—September 26, 2006

Today Patricia, a CNA who had been away from work for a long time due to an on-the-job injury, came in to see me. Apparently, her lawyer advised her to explore the possibility of being accommodated in some job here. Before her injury, Patricia had worked here for 13 years.

When she arrived, everyone seemed very happy to see her. Clearly, she was a joy to work with. She had a beautiful smile, and you could see she was a people person. I imagine she had been an excellent CNA.

She told me her hands are almost useless to her now because her wrists are in constant pain. "I could feel it getting worse and worse every year I worked here," she said. "All the pulling and lifting we were doing all the time. After a while, I just could not take the pain anymore. The surgery did not seem to help at all. I feel useless."

Tears welled up in her eyes when she said, "My daughter just had her first baby. My first grandchild . . . and I can't even hold him."

She continued, "This job got me off welfare. If I could work I would. Some people are trying to make it seem as if I am making this up because I don't want to work. And that couldn't be further from the truth. I want to work but I can't. My hands don't work."

I really didn't know what to say. I felt terrible for her.

According to Occupational Safety and Health Administration (OSHA) statistics, working as a CNA in a nursing home is one of the three or so most hazardous occupations in the nation. Many people don't realize just how dangerous it is. Many CNAs have no choice but to work through the pain, day in and day out, after an injury, since many lack basic health insurance and paid time off benefits.

Patricia and I knew that we could not accommodate her because we didn't have any jobs that didn't require use of her hands. I thanked her for coming in and wished her luck. When I reached my hand toward her, she pulled hers away and said, "Sorry, it hurts too much to shake your hand." She held her hands limply together as she walked out of my office looking down. I followed her but she left too quickly.

Day 111—September 29, 2006

After three months on the job, we've had some significant accomplishments.

Quality of Work Life Measures

- Annualized nursing staff turnover rate over the past three months (July, August, and September) is 35%, down from 77% over the previous 12 months (July 2005–June 2006).
- We're on course for lowering our employee terminations from about 70 a year to 32. Given that it costs us about $2,000 to replace an employee, this represents a savings of about $76,000.
- We had eight full-time vacant positions in the nursing department on June 12, 2006. On August 15th, that number was reduced to 0. On September 1, we established a waiting list of CNAs who want to work here.

- The nursing department's overtime hours declined from an average of 1,400 hours a month in March, April, and May to 550 hours in September.
- The nursing staff has worked short staffed (with less than the optimal number of staff) on just one shift and in just one neighborhood over the past 30 days.
- Call-outs from nursing department staff, which totaled 52 this past April, declined to an average of 32 a month in June, July, and August.

Clinical Measures

- From January through May, we used physical restraints on an average of 63% of the residents. That dropped to a monthly average of 37% from June through September. September's rate was the best yet, at just 16%.
- We averaged 14.2 resident falls a month from January through May. From June through September, that dropped to a monthly average of 9, including just 7 in September.
- The percentage of residents who developed pressure ulcers while here declined from an average of 5.9% to 3.5% in September.

Business Measures

- The average daily occupancy rate for the month of September 2006 is the highest it has ever been in the past five years.
- The average daily Medicare occupancy rate for the month of September is the 7th highest it has ever been in the past five years.
- The average profit margin was 15% (November 2005–May 2006). Over the past three months (June, July, and August 2006) the average profit margin increased to 21.3%.

I knew that once we stabilized our staffing, our care would improve and that would bring in more residents. The combination of stable staffing and higher census gives us the business gains. Of course, sustaining and building on these gains will be the true test of deep change. But the preliminary results look pretty good. Things really seemed to come together in September. It looks like a breakthrough month. The "flywheel" is spinning faster, and the cumulative effect of all the earlier changes in the same direction is paying off.

Day 114—October 2, 2006

It was not a good day.

One of our newer CNAs, Dolmi, reported that a veteran CNA, Lisa, was kicking one of the residents yesterday while the resident was suspended in the air, held up by a Hoyer lift.

She was explaining the situation to Andy when I walked in. "She seemed so angry," Dolmi said. "I was scared of her face. I couldn't sleep last night."

I asked her to start over for me and be very specific.

She said, "I was helping Lisa transfer a resident using a Hoyer lift when the resident started to sway. I was trying to steady the resident when Lisa became very angry and started kicking her. I was so scared. Lisa was so mad. I know it's my obligation to report this." Tears started to flow down her cheeks.

Then she said, "I don't want Lisa to know that I reported her. I am afraid."

Then Andy said, "This is confidential. We appreciate you telling us. Thank you very much. Thank you. I will come by to speak with you later. Please let me have a minute with Mr. David." And she stepped away.

I shut the door and said, "This is not good. We need to do a full investigation. Have you ever had any other reports about Lisa?"

Andy said, "I have only heard that, in general, the staff can be a little rough on Station Four. But I have not had any specific complaints about Lisa. No."

I said, "I need you to complete a full body check on the resident. Do you have the policy on reporting abuse?"

He gave me the file containing the forms and the policy. Before leaving his office, I asked him to let me know if the resident had suffered any trauma.

This is rough. Physical abuse! The residents on Station Four are tough to care for. Many are severely debilitated and physically or verbally abusive to the staff. It's the kind of environment where I could imagine a staff member losing patience with a resident. But from what Dolmi described, this alleged abuse was unprovoked.

Andy suspects there is no truth to these accusations, but I believe that something did occur. We may never know for sure.

I made the report to the DHS. First I called and then I faxed over the completed form. Then I felt pretty lousy about it the rest of the day and well into the night.

I got home and wanted to escape from the thoughts of work. What can I do to stop thinking about work? I bet many administrators want to forget work for awhile. I know I do.

Day 115—October 3, 2006

The Quality Campaign for Nursing Home Excellence was launched last Friday in Washington, D.C. I would have liked to have been there, but I felt far away from all the glamour and hype of the next big push to improve America's nursing homes.

I was lost in the thick of just trying to manage one of the over 16,000 nursing homes nationwide, oblivious to the speeches of people standing at podiums and saying that administrators like me need to buckle down and improve quality. The only reason I even knew about the campaign launch is because I stay connected to the national nursing home news through a service provided by the American Health Care Association, the trade association my facility belongs to.

I believe that the typical administrator feels as disconnected as I do from the national nursing home news and quality campaigns such as this one. Most of us are just trying to get through the day, day after day after day. The podium is far away from the nurses' station. The speeches aren't heard in these halls.

Are you calling to me from Washington, D.C.? What are you asking me to do?

Our trade association's fights on Capitol Hill are far, far away, not like our fights with the old clothes dryer that just broke down again on a Friday night as we were all trying to go home after a rough week. And national campaigns to improve quality don't feel all that urgent here. Fixing the dryer does.

Are you speaking to me? I think I'm in charge of one of the nursing homes you're speaking about at the podium in Washington, D.C. I'm right here.

Day 116—October 4, 2006

Still working on that abuse case. Things like this take up a tremendous amount of time, and my to-do list keeps getting longer and longer. What gets pushed to the side is the work I need to do to move the organization forward. It's frustrating for me. Bogged down in this while the flywheel doesn't get a push.

It's still hard to imagine this abuse happening. I was certainly hoping to find out today that Lisa could totally negate the story with credible witnesses. She completely denied ever interacting with Dolmi on the morning of the alleged incident.

So we have two CNAs telling completely different stories. I asked Andy, "What are you thinking about this now? Which way are you leaning?"

Andy responded, "I think something must have happened. Lisa is an intimidating person who has been here for awhile. Why would Dolmi, who is pretty passive, accuse her unless something really occurred? They have no bad blood between them. I told Lisa it doesn't look good for her unless she can produce a credible witness who can negate Dolmi's story."

Lisa did pull in another CNA, a brand new CNA named Oda who was in orientation over the past weekend. Lisa explained that Oda had helped her transfer the resident at the time Dolmi says that she was assisting Lisa. However, Oda could not remember assisting Lisa with that particular resident. He said he helped a lot of people that day. He felt bad that he couldn't help Lisa by agreeing with her statements, but he was being honest.

As an organization, we are stuck. If we fire Lisa, she has a solid wrongful termination case against us. If we don't fire her, we may be exposing vulnerable residents to someone who may have abused a resident—and exposing ourselves to possible repercussions from the DHS.

I feel the sheer weight of the decision, and the consequences of the decision for everyone involved. In my gut, right now, I know I'm responsible for protecting people. And I feel in my gut that Lisa may have the potential to abuse a resident. She has been known to scream and curse. She could cross the line to physical abuse.

It's better for her to move on. We cannot confirm that the incident did not occur, and I must protect the residents. That's my main concern.

This job can sure wear me out. I am so emotionally drained by this I can't feel anything right now. I'm just numb.

Day 117—October 5, 2006

There have been many twists and turns with the abuse case. Today, there was another turn that took us down a whole new path.

The accuser, Dolmi, was apparently talking about the case this morning. According to a few witnesses, she confronted Sanjila and demanded that she back up her statements. But Sanjila did just the opposite. She said that it was Dolmi, not Lisa, who was of questionable character. Now Dolmi's behavior is leading me to question her whole story.

Dolmi rambles on and on and on when she talks. She is absolutely exhausting to listen to. She jumps from one subject to another. And she speaks very fast in a heavy accent. The more I listen to her, the more inconsistencies I find in her story. She may not be mentally stable.

This is becoming more and more complicated each day. This is a tough call.[3]

Day 135—October 23, 2006

Charge nurses with poor supervisory skills can, and do, undermine management's efforts to retain and engage the best CNAs. In the final analysis, the charge nurse is the CNA's supervisor, and bad supervision can drive away a good worker.

Today, the staffing coordinator, Kris, informed me that one of our best new CNAs, Julie, is asking to be placed on call rather than work a full schedule. When I asked why Julie had changed her mind, Kris said, "She said she wants to spend more time with her daughter."

I was distraught. She had only been with us a few months, but Julie was doing a great job. I suspected there was something more to her request to go on call. After all, when I interviewed her she had clearly indicated that she wanted and needed a full-time job.

In the late afternoon, I walked by Andy's office. He looked upset, lifting his glasses off of the bridge of his nose and rubbing his eyes. I stepped into his office and saw that he was talking to Julie. Andy said, "Mr. David, please close the door."

After I shut the door Andy said, "Julie, please tell Mr. David what you were just saying to me."

Julie explained that her charge nurse, Dolores, is very rude to her and the rest of the CNAs. She said Dolores orders them around and does not bother to call them by their names. She said Dolores speaks harshly in a military way. Julie said, "It makes me feel bad to come to work."

I said, "Is this why you asked to be put on call?"

Julie nodded her head yes.

Andy said, "Please never let these things sit for so long. Come to see me." He gave Julie his cell phone number and promised to talk to Dolores. "If I can change her behavior toward you and the rest of the CNAs, will you stay with us full time?" he asked.

"Yes. I will stay full time," said Julie.

It just goes to show that for the CNAs, it's all about their relationship with their immediate supervisor. It doesn't matter how they feel about me or Andy. What matters is how they get along with the charge nurse—their boss.

I resolve to focus on educating the charge nurses about the critical role they play in retaining and respecting our CNAs.

Day 136—October 24, 2006

We got softer toilet paper.

Chris, the new housekeeping supervisor (who is doing a great job), came to me and asked if we wanted to get a higher grade of toilet paper. I was struck by what a smart idea that was. I said, "Sure," and it was done. We went from buying the cheapest, roughest, thinnest toilet paper to a softer, higher-quality, two-ply brand.

I got to thinking about the symbolism around this act of buying better toilet paper. I remember Dr. Bill Thomas, who founded the Eden Alternative, talking about some nursing home owners and administrators whose decisions reflect a stingy mindset, and the negative effect that can have on an organization. His words ring true to me as I look at the cheap toilet paper we were buying. It was one step up from a leaf.

Purchasing softer toilet paper is now one of the key changes we have made here in our attempts to deinstitutionalize the environment. Softer toilet paper is now symbolic of our "softer" environment and our "softer" approach with the staff. The investment in better toilet paper is an investment in human comfort. It shouts, in a very basic way: "We care about you!"

Our residents, and the people who work here, deserve softer, higher-quality toilet paper. It costs a little bit more, but it's worth it. The people here are worth it.

Day 137—October 25, 2006

I am driving Charlo, my central supply person, crazy. I consistently ask the staff what they need and they tell me. Then I go to Charlo to fulfill their requests.

I know this will result in better care. In addition, I realize how important it is to demonstrate that I care and I am really listening to the staff and acting on their suggestions. There is an organizational, a scientific, and a psychological benefit to asking them what they want and then delivering on it.

The first request I received was for bendable straws. Straight straws make drinking difficult for residents who are lying flat. A bendable straw allows residents to drink when they want to and allows caregivers to assist residents with less struggle. Again, it costs a little more, but they're worth it, and it creates efficiencies for the staff and reduces dependencies of the residents. Everyone wins and everyone's happier.

After we got the bendable straws, the requests for all types of supplies started. And I started to drive Charlo crazy.

Day 142—October 30, 2006

I am perplexed by the "it's strictly business" approach of many of the corporate staff. It seems to me that earlier in my career, I heard more about the "quality of care" side of the business. But now, all they seem to react to is business data.

Two weeks ago, I shared two pieces of bad news with my boss. One was about the potential write-off of $12,000 due to an error we made regarding a Medicare Part A denial notice. The other was the accusation of physical abuse by one CNA against another. Well, over these past two weeks, my boss has inquired about the potential $12,000 write-off five times—four times via email and once in a voice message. Meanwhile, the abuse report seems to have slipped his mind. He has never once inquired about it.

That speaks to where the focus of the company really is. I am disappointed that I am not seeing a genuine focus on the residents or the staff. There is a lot of pressure to keep occupancy high and overtime low, and nothing else seems to matter right now.

The budget process has been a sham. Last week they said the budgets need to be done ASAP. I received some information on Wednesday that had a turnaround response time of 9:00 a.m. the next day. When I asked about the cut they proposed of three licensed nurses and three CNAs a day, they responded with sarcasm and a comparison between their proposed hours PPD and the "industry standard."

"Industry standard"—why would anyone want to benchmark their data against an obsolete industry standard? Isn't that "standard" one that the general public wants to avoid?

I do not want to cut even one hour from our daily nursing hours. In fact, I want to add more staff and hours. A cut of six staff per day is absolutely insane. It would bring the flywheel to a halt.

Andy and I both offered to eliminate our budgeted, full-time assistant positions (assistant DON and assistant administrator) in order to keep our current nursing staff levels. The salaries of those two positions would cover at least three CNAs and one licensed nurse. We both agree that having enough frontline staff is more important than hiring additional department heads, although I would really like to see Andy keep the assistant DON position and find someone great to fill it.

Day 143—October 31, 2006

The Halloween party was a huge hit with the residents and staff today. For me, Halloween has always been a great opportunity to create laughter and some fun in a nursing home. Because of the spirit of the people here, I had a feeling this one would be great. And it was.

I encouraged the staff to dress up by offering cash prizes for best costume—$100 first place, $60 second place, $30 third place. As a result, we had great participation and some very creative costumes. The residents were the judges, and they were the only ones who could vote.

I dressed up like a woman. I got my entire costume from the lost and found—which is really just a huge pile of unmarked clothes in the far corner of the laundry. Hector, the laundry aide, looked at me as if I were crazy when I started holding up dresses to see if they would fit. "So now you know the truth about me," I joked. "So what? Just don't tell anyone, Hector!"

He shook his head and walked away with a wide grin.

I pulled out the biggest bra in the pile and stuffed it with a bunch of socks. My mother was visiting, and she brought a great wig, which I put on. After getting dressed in the privacy of my office, I called out to Vicky, the activity assistant. She came over to help.

"Please put some makeup on me," I asked.

She couldn't stop laughing. She kept looking at my big chest. I may have overdone it with the size of the bra this year.

Finally, she got hold of herself and completed my makeup, and I was ready for "prime time." I just loved to see the faces of the residents, staff, and visitors when they saw me in my costume. People were cracking up. They loved seeing me let my guard down and make some fun of myself.

We had a great party. The karaoke really adds a lot to the spirit of the group. Some of the staff sang a song or two. At one point, the entire roomful of 40 residents and 35 staff members were singing and clapping together to the song, "We Are Family." I was overwhelmed with emotion by the sight and sound of it. I sat down and just took it all in. For that fleeting moment, we were "family," and we all felt it. There was love in that room. It felt amazing.

Halloween—what a great holiday. And what an opportunity to build the spirit of community.

Day 154—November 11, 2006

Today, I took my turn as "weekend manager" on a Saturday. It was rainy and cloudy—a strange weather day for California, where it never seems to rain. But today it poured.

Yesterday was payday. Historically, there were always a lot of call-offs on both Saturday and Sunday after payday, but there were no call-offs today. Clearly, the tide is turning. I will make sure to share that with the staff. I need to publicly talk about this change in our culture. By publicly acknowledging the improved weekend attendance I will be reinforcing that positive behavior.

Without all of the usual interruptions that come on a weekday, I finally had time to unpack the eight boxes of files I had lugged across the country. The boxes are full of my favorite articles, research studies, and books, as well as staff turnover data, QIO learning materials, and PowerPoint presentations. Every year, I add more material.

In my office, there is a large, green metal cabinet with three drawers packed full of sad, bad stories of surveys and visits from DHS. There are thick files filled with poor survey results and the plans of correction that accompany them. And there are overflowing files from single inspections triggered by complaints that look like they took up a lot of the administrator's time. Every one of the files contains a story. Some of the ones I looked at are nightmares.

For two hours, as I replaced the files in the green cabinet with files from my boxes, I realized that the knowledge in my files could actually have prevented the bad inspection results documented in the other files I was removing. If only this organization had implemented the evidence-based strategies contained in my files, they would have had far fewer files crammed with paperwork from poor inspections. It's ironic.

Day 158—November 15, 2006

Today I received the certified financial officer's (CFO's) email answer to my question about canceling the EAP as an employee benefit. The contract is up for renewal, and the CFO wants to save some money by letting it lapse. He said he asked my former assistant administrator, Liz, about this a few months ago. "She said it wasn't being used, so it can be canceled with no consequences."

I responded, "Liz did not know how to use it. The EAP is a very effective program and we plan on using it. In fact, we may already have saved one CNA by referring her to the EAP. Since she called the EAP her attendance has improved and she looks better.

"It costs us about $2,000 to replace a CNA," I added. "If we use the EAP to save just four CNAs a year, the program pays for itself."

He said, "None of the other facilities have it. To tell you the truth, I am not even sure what it is. But we need to cut it out of the budget. In fact, we already have."

I responded, "We employ the working poor. The EAP helps employees solve dilemmas in their home life, allowing them to be engaged staff members. We should not cancel the employee assistance program. I know how to use it so that we will get a return on this investment. Please, do not cancel it."

Nursing homes all over the country should be signing up for EAP benefits for their staff. The perfect formula to boost loyalty and reduce turnover is as follows:

EAP + *no-fault attendance policy* + *paid time off* = *loyalty and low rates of absenteeism*

Under our no-fault attendance policy, call-offs are simply counted, not qualified according to how legitimate some manager deems the call-out excuse to be. If the staff know that all call-offs will be treated the same regardless of the reason for the call-off, staff are more inclined to tell the truth about why they are calling off. And as managers get more of the truth from the staff, they can easily make referrals to the EAP when appropriate, so trained professionals can help the staff member and, many times, turn their attendance issue around.

Unfortunately, our CFO's reaction is the norm in long-term care, where the mandate is to cut costs wherever you can. It's all about "make the financials look better this month—and do it fast."

Day 159—November 16, 2006

Mr. Waitts turned 82 today, and he sure felt special: It seemed just about everyone wished him a happy birthday. That's because we've started honoring residents on their birthday in two ways—if they agree to it. One is that we tie balloons to their wheelchair on their birthday. The other is we give them a cupcake and sing Happy Birthday to them after lunch.

The balloons make it so easy for the staff to recognize whose birthday it is and wish them a happy birthday. But also, our environment and culture have shifted enough that peers encourage each other to do so. The staff are just plain nice people whose natural impulse is to celebrate people's birthdays. They just need to know when they are. And this system alerts them.

A system to make it easy for staff to see whose birthday it is combined with the right people being employed here, who are naturally inclined to honor others' birthdays, results in—wow—the right people doing the right things under the right conditions. When it all comes together, it's a beautiful thing.

Mr. Waitts felt so good on his birthday today.

He felt loved.

Day 160—November 17, 2006

Diana was singing this afternoon. As I made my way through Station Four, along came Diana. She was singing and she didn't stop.

This was the same Diana who had looked like a wreck four weeks ago. After counseling her about her attendance, which was becoming spotty, Andy and I had learned of her struggles to raise two kids while clearing only $1,200 a month and paying $900 in rent. She looked thin and haggard and appeared tired all the time. It had been reported that she was found sleeping in a resident's closet.

But today, she was singing. She had a smile on her face, which looked fuller than it had before. She looked well rested and happy.

I followed her into a resident's room and said, "Your singing sounds great. I am so glad to hear you singing."

She just smiled.

We really helped her. Not just by helping her apply for food stamps and insisting that she call the EAP for guidance. And arranging for her rent to be reduced, as Andy somehow managed to do.

We also helped her on a much deeper level, by showing that we cared about her as a person. We demonstrated that we wanted her to succeed on the job and in life. I think Diana really needed that. It feels so good to see her with some self-esteem.

I rode the elevator down with Diana when her shift ended at 3 p.m. She told me she was coming in to work tomorrow—on her day off. In other words, she's gone from frequent call-offs to picking up extra shifts.

It's amazing what caring for people can do for them—and for your organization.

Day 165—November 22, 2006

I was so proud last night. I completed a set of thorough rounds throughout the facility from 9:45 to 10:30 p.m. The residents looked well cared for, the facility looked clean and tidy, and the staff seemed calm and attentive. There were no call bells ringing. The place really looked good.

About five or six CNAs gathered around me to talk in the hall. I said, "I want you to know that the residents look well cared for tonight. You are all really doing an excellent job. I can see that you are taking good care of the residents and I really appreciate it."

They just smiled and nodded. A few blushed.

Caregivers are such good people. I am finding that as the culture and climate are enhanced here, each staff member's best character traits seem to flourish and go on display more often. Relationships grow strong and positive in cultures where people display their best qualities. Communication is easy and accurate when relationships are solid.

It starts with reducing the stress—which brings out the worst in people. There is so much we have done to reduce stress for the staff here. Human beings under stress tend to display their weakest character traits. In the past three months, our staff have had to work short just three times. Eliminating short staffing has done a lot to diminish people's stress levels, allowing these wonderful, caring people to be at their best.

I was really proud of the staff here last night. And I made sure to tell them so.

Day 168—November 25, 2006

I have been writing less lately. I think a lot of it has to do with things around here becoming routine for me. I am less amazed by all that's going on around me than I was when I first arrived. I guess that is to be expected.

Also, things have gotten calmer here, so there's less "shock and awe."

It's not so strange for me here anymore. I am not "taken aback" like I often was five months ago. I hope that's not a sign that I am becoming complacent . . . or worse yet, reinstitutionalized.

I still get overwhelmed sometimes. This job is so demanding. It is very difficult to concentrate on anything for an extended period of time. I feel compelled to get out of my office as often as I can, so I can see what's going on. I try to stay positive and consistent.

Whenever I have been in the office for a couple of hours, I get curious about how things are going in the neighborhoods. Then I get up and make rounds.

By now, I know everyone's name and something about him or her. The staff is very friendly to me. This is quite a change from when I first arrived. I see a lot of smiles and frequently hear laughter in the courtyard or in the neighborhoods. It's nice.

It's evident that the culture is much better than it used to be. You can see it, hear it, and feel it. When I remember how it was just five months ago, I feel good. I know the residents are getting better care and service.

Day 173—November 30, 2006

November has been another record-setting month. We averaged 116.75 residents per day, the highest occupancy number in five years by a hefty margin, and that included by far the most Medicare Part A residents in that same five-year span.

But what I was really proud of today was the weekly pressure ulcer report. Our in-house acquired pressure ulcer rate dropped to 2.5%.

When I was handed the report, I immediately noticed how short the list was. I was used to seeing almost a full page of names of residents who had pressure sores. But today, the list took up only about a third of a page.

I said to Andy, "I loved that pressure ulcer report today. That looks really good. Excellent work."

He said, "I know. I couldn't believe it. I had to check for myself to confirm it. So I did. But it's accurate."

"That's excellent. And we took care of so many residents. What a great month!" I responded with a huge smile.

Andy was beaming too.

Day 179—December 6, 2006

I am still amazed at how fast the time goes when I'm working at the nursing home. I feel stressed by the lack of resident contact and conversation. It's strange that I feel so busy, yet can't find the time for the most important people.

As I stopped in the hallway outside Mr. Waitts's room today, I thought: "It's 2:00, he is my neighbor, and I have not seen him all day." I felt guilty and sad.

He was leaning way over in a dark room, trying to figure something out. I knocked, he looked up, and I walked in and said, "Do you mind if I turn on some lights?"

He said, "Lights! I was just trying to save you some money."

I responded, "Don't worry about that. You need to see what you are doing. . . . What are you doing?"

"I'm trying to turn on this radio," he said. Clearly, he was frustrated.

I found the switch and turned it on. Then Mr. Waitts said, "Where have you been today? Your door's been open but you ain't been in there."

He had noticed: I was there, but I was not there for him. Where are my priorities right now? What's wrong with me? When can I carve out some time to see the people who live here? I am so focused on the workers I am not seeing the residents enough. This has to change.

"I know," I mumbled, "I have been downstairs all day leading an orientation because our staff developer is out ill and I had this report due and. . . . "

He smiled and said, "You're busy. I know. I see things. I don't waste my time watching TV. I watch everything and I'm watching you. You got more plants too. I see that! You're getting so many plants you can't keep track of 'em. And don't leave poor Ruth to water all those plants. She can't carry that heavy water jug around here."

"I know. . . . I won't. I'll water the plants today. Don't worry about it." I said.

After a long pause I said, "You'll see more of me tomorrow."

"I hope so." said Mr. Waitts. Then he repeated, "I hope so."

He always finds a way to slow me down, in a good way.

Day 181—December 8, 2006

I am determined to get the CNA peer mentor program off the ground. It seems to be coming together. We have seven committed CNAs who are willing to step up and model what a great caregiver is all about. They will orient new staff to their consistent assignment within their neighborhoods, convey important information to their teammates, and take the pressure off busy charge nurses.

We had the interested CNAs formally apply for the peer mentor positions and I was so moved by what the applicants wrote in their peer mentor application essays. They clearly are striving to do their best and give compassionate care. They all said that they love their job—and the residents.

I have had a couple of meetings with them. I really enjoy the opportunity to speak with a small group of committed individuals like these CNAs. So far, we have focused on the process of welcoming and educating new staff to their neighborhoods. Also, we spent a considerable amount of time at the last meeting discussing the need for peer mentors to socially support new staff members, reaching out to them for as long as six months after their date of hire.

Next week, we will share the data from each of the different neighborhoods with the peer mentors. I will highlight the quality measures they can influence most. These individuals are like sponges. They are extremely bright.

I see CNAs as intelligent professionals who just have not been afforded the same opportunities as others. Lazy? Hardly. Dimwitted? Absolutely not! Unskilled labor? No way!

All of the peer mentors were given a 25-cent-an-hour raise for their efforts. On the same day I was completing their paperwork for the pay increase, two of our best CNAs approached me and Andy about an increase in pay. Both deserved it, and they were only making the minimum CNA hourly rate of $11 per hour.

I couldn't make them peer mentors, since they didn't have enough experience, and I cannot approve raises except on the anniversary of someone's hiring. I had a dilemma. So, I slipped their names in with the list of peer mentors that went to payroll that week. They were not going to work as a peer mentor, but no one would know that but me.

I asked Andy to tell them about the increase. And after he did, both came to see me.

"I am so grateful," said Olessi. "Thank you."

Nama said, "I just want to say that you listened to me. That was so nice. I really appreciate it."

"You deserve it, you both deserve it." I said. "You are doing a great job."

They both smiled broadly and stepped out of my office respectfully. They both paused at the door and gave me a long look. I looked up at them, they nodded and stepped out.

Day 181—December 9th, 2006

I just completed an analysis of the data to see how far we have come. I am constantly looking at the data. It's not enough to do it once. I do it all the time—how are we doing? What do the data tell us? We're making gains and sustaining them. Here are the results today:

Accomplishments—6 Months

Quality of Work Life Key Measures:

- Annualized nursing staff turnover rate is getting better. Now we're at 28% over the past six months (June–November) compared to 35% three months ago, and 77% turnover rate over the previous 12 months (July 2005–June 2006).
  – The CNA turnover rate has declined from 94% to 38%.
  – The licensed nurses turnover rate declined from 43% to 7%.
- Still no nursing department vacancies, and we still have a waiting list.
- The nursing department's overtime hours are down even more. From an average of 1,400 hours per month in March, April, and May 2006 to 550 in September, and now, the new three-month average is 450 hours for September, October, and November 2006.
- The nursing staff has only been short staffed (worked with less than the optimal number of staff) on three occasions in the past 100 days (September–December 10, 2006), less than one per month.
- The nursing department staff call-offs holding steady at an average of 32 call-offs per month over the past 6 months (June–November) after a total of 52 times in April 2006.

Key Clinical Measures:

- Resident falls declined from a monthly average of 14.2 falls per month from January through May 2006 to a monthly average of 11 falls per month from June through November 2006.
- The percentage of residents with in-house-acquired pressure ulcers has declined from an average of 5.9% to 3.4% (September–November).

Business Measures:

- The average daily occupancy rate of 116.6 for the month of November 2006 is the highest average daily occupancy rate compared to any month looking back over the past five years (60 months).
- The average daily Medicare occupancy rate of 16.5 for the month of November is the highest average compared to any month over the past five years.
- The average profit margin was 15% (November 2005–May 2006). Over the past three months (September–November 2006) the average profit margin increased to 23.7%.

Day 185—December 12, 2006

It looks like we are going to lose Diana after all. She is the CNA Andy and I helped a few months ago. She called off again on Saturday, right after payday. It's a shame.

I was so hopeful that she was better after we helped her. She seemed happy for about five weeks. But then the pattern started again. She started coming late and then calling off. She has lots of reasons why she has to call off. Her life seems very chaotic, out of control, and inconsistent.

Diana says she is moving back home with her mother, who lives in Redding, California.

We did what we could for her. We were patient and kind. We showed we cared about her as a person. Oh well . . . maybe next time. . . .

Day 186—December 13, 2006

Meeting with the CNA peer mentors gives me a wonderful opportunity to learn what I need to focus on. I enjoy talking to our brightest, most committed caregivers.

This is an opportunity that few leaders create for themselves. And yet everything I have read about leadership says regularly meeting with those doing the work is critical to organizational success.

Today was our first "official" CNA peer mentor meeting, and it did not go as expected. I didn't even look at my agenda, since the peer mentors led the discussion. I guess that's how it should be. They know what needs to be talked about.

It started with Natasha letting off some steam. "I was pretty angry this morning, and it takes a lot to get me mad," she said.

"Why?" I asked.

"There just was not any linen or Depends anywhere. I can't do my job without the basics. That's never happened to me before here. It's frustrating!" She said. She sure looked frustrated.

Others chimed in: "It was rough. When Charlo in central supply goes on vacation this always happens. She needs help. It's not her fault," said Gene in a loud voice.

"I do not know what happens with the towels," Tessie added. "It just seems like we never have enough. We always run out."

"I thought we had this solved," I said. "We spend about $850 on new linen each month. This is a problem that we can solve. I will get a bunch of linen out there. I want to see our linen closets full. I am sorry about this."

I am frustrated. I feel like I am failing them if they do not have the basic supplies to do their job. I need to get them the supplies.

I did as I said. I called the housekeeping supervisor, Chris, and asked to get all the new linen out in circulation. Then I advised him to purchase over $1,200 in new linen.

Day 194—December 21, 2006

A few days ago I noticed one of the CNAs on the day shift who usually works on Rockridge Station, Sarina, passionately admiring a candle set her co-worker had won at the raffle we held at the community meeting earlier in the week. She seemed to really love the candle set. So today, when I went shopping for presents for the night shift's community meeting, I picked up the same candle set.

I saw her in the dining room and walked right up and handed her a bag with the candle set in it. "Merry Christmas, Sarina!" I said.

She looked inside and a wide grin came over her face. She said, "This is the one I wanted. Thank you so much. This is the one I wanted."

I recently read a book about retaining staff, and one principle really stood out for me: retention is an individual activity. It may seem risky to give a gift to an individual employee. After all, some of the employees might see this as special treatment. But I would do it for them too. So I'll take that risk.

One of the best parts about being a nursing home administrator are moments like these, when you can reach out to someone like Sarina. She appears so tough on the outside. But she needs positive acknowledgment as much as anyone. And this small investment may lead to her being completely engaged.

Day 198—December 25, 2006

I knocked and entered Mr. Waitts's room around 4:30 p.m. Our exchange went the way it usually does at that time of day.

I said, "Can I turn on your light for you, sir? It's dark in here."

"I thought you didn't want me to turn it on to save money," he said.

"I don't want you sitting in the dark," I replied, flipping on the light.

He was facing the sliding glass doors, looking through partially open blinds at the Christmas lights glittering in the tree in the courtyard. I stepped over and opened the drapes some more. It was Christmas Day, and it looked like it.

Mr. Waitts and the rest of the residents had just enjoyed a great meal, and it was time for me to get home to my wife and our daughter, Isabella.

As I started for the door, Mr. Waitts said: "Nobody's ever cared for me like you do."

That was a great gift for me today.

Day 201—December 28, 2006

Andy was pretty upset about a resident we admitted yesterday who died three hours after the admission. He felt that this was a "dump," where the hospital was just trying to avoid counting the man in their mortality statistics, so they sent him to us to die.

I feel pretty down about the whole thing too. This happens sometimes, and it stinks.

Day 215—January 11, 2007

I've noticed that people will step up when you create the right climate for them. Families and residents are noticing how nice the staff is now. People can feel the positive employee morale that is building here. I can feel it too.

The new staff are doing an excellent job. People of good character do the right thing in the right way at the right time without a lot of oversight or supervision or policies. Simply, good people do well. Our hiring decisions and supportive management policies are paying off, and the elders are benefiting.

I feel good because the facility has never been so clean, the staff are happy and the data are really looking great.

I love the people who work here.

Day 228—January 24, 2007

Today, we had our most effective process improvement meeting since my arrival. A lot of that was thanks to our medical director, Dr. Mitchell.

The doctor told our department heads they were the best ones we've ever had. "We are on the verge of reaching the next level," he said. "We need to pick a few key clinical indicators and focus on improving them. Let's not bite off too much. But let's really focus on the ones we choose."

It was music to my ears. The research-based evidence is clear—an active, engaged medical director can have an enormous positive impact on a nursing home. Dr. Mitchell is a geriatrician and certified by the American Medical Directors Association. I could not be happier that he is a part of our organization.

We looked at our quality indicators to see what needed improvement most. The six-month trend report showed drastic improvements in our clinical outcomes. Certainly, there are areas that we need to focus on, but overall the data look darn good.

I said to the group, "Our data show that not only do we do a good job of preventing pressure ulcers, but when we admit residents who already have pressure ulcers, we heal them within 90 days. We should be very proud of that."

They all clapped.

Day 239—February 4, 2007

On Friday, I was asked at a meeting if I had any announcements to make. Only one came to mind.

One of our housekeepers, Maria, had told me that another housekeeper, Lillian, was not at our last community meeting, where we talked about how to pack up a resident's belongings after a death. After the mortuary took away the body of one of our residents who had passed away, Lillian put her belongings in a trash bag and placed it on the bed. "The CNAs told Lillian that this was not the way we treated our deceased residents' belongings anymore," Maria told me. "The belongings are to be carefully and respectfully packed up in boxes. You see, Mr. David, we listen to what you say."

This may sound like a small victory, but it was an important one. Sometimes I get so caught up in trying to fix what isn't working that I miss moments like these. Lately, I have been focused on an anonymous staff member who has been defacing the memos and notes that I have been hanging in the back service elevator.

Elevators are a great place to post information for staff, since they have nothing to do while riding in the elevator but read what's been posted on the wall. But twice now, someone has defaced the community's mission statement that I hung up there.

The second time it happened, I removed postings he or she had slashed with a knife and put up a note asking him or her to stop. That note was slashed too, so I left the bulletin board bare for a day.

I felt very low. This makes an already tough job even tougher. I begin to question my own abilities as a leader. I ask myself, "Who I am kidding?"

It helps that many staff members have been watching this transpire and have been very supportive. "I hope you find the person doing that. It is so childish," said Albert, the dietary aide. Dave, the housekeeper, said: "I hope you find that person." And Charlo, the central supply clerk, suggested putting my postings in a glass display case so the person can't get to them.

In front of the small group that had gathered around us, I answered: "That's a great idea Charlo, but I want our culture to prevail here. I want the individual to have access to the postings and decide to stop. I want the person to stop doing it because that's the right thing to do."

I went on to say, "Our culture is winning out. Just last week, the CNAs trained a housekeeper to stop packing up a deceased resident's belongings in a plastic trash bag. They explained to her that the new way is to carefully and respectfully place the items in boxes. So, you see, that's a sure sign that our culture is getting healthy, and the same thing can happen here. Let's give it a chance. But thank you for your support."

Day 242—February 7, 2007

Last night, I felt better after a long talk with my wife about the person defacing the notes in the elevator. She said, "Don't take it too personally. The individual who is doing this is disrespecting everyone who lives and works there—not just you. When the other staff see defaced memos in an organization, it brings the whole place down." My wife is very wise.

I decided to appeal once more to the person who is defacing my notes. This morning, I posted the following notice in the back elevator:

Attention: To the Individual Who Keeps Defacing My Postings Here

My wife explained to me last night that I was taking this too personally. She said that when you deface the postings here, you are disrespecting our entire community and everyone who lives and works here.

These postings are meant to remind us that what we are doing here is noble and quite remarkable. The postings are intended to inspire us to strive to treat the residents here with dignity and respect and love.

So . . . stop defacing the postings here.

Next to it, I posted:

Love cures people.
Both the ones who give love and the ones who receive it.

Day 244—February 9, 2007

Jay is an older African American male and a native of our city who just got certified as a nursing assistant and is looking for his first job as a CNA. He looks as if he has had some rough times in his life, but he is well dressed and polite. I interviewed him, just like everyone else who fills out an application. After three weeks and no word back from me, Jay reappeared and asked that a copy of his CPR card be included with his application.

While he was waiting, I watched him politely open a door for someone pushing a resident in a wheelchair. I was impressed by that action; he anticipated a need and acted, so I decided I needed to speak to him again.

We had a conversation as I was picking up cigarette butts out of the ground cover in the front of the facility. A daily chore of mine. "Why should I hire you?" I asked.

Jay said, "Because I will not let you down. I am very eager to work. I have had some issues in the past but now I am responsible for my three-year-old girl." He pulled out her picture from his wallet and I looked at it. I have a beautiful three-year-old daughter myself.

I looked closely at Jay. He was well groomed. He looked right back into my eyes. He looked sincere and determined. He really wanted a job and a chance.

"A lot of people apply here. I only hire people of good character. Will you respect the elders?" I asked. I started picking up the butts again.

"I won't let you down," he said. "I am a good person. And yes, I treat elderly people like my grandparents."

We hired him that day, just last Monday. Today, Friday, Andy came in to my office and said that the background check on Jay had come back and it wasn't good.

The report listed three felonies. One was drunk driving, another was selling drugs, and the third was for disorderly conduct. All told, he had spent 122 days in jail, all in 2001.

"Did he reveal this in the interview?" I asked.

"Yes, he did. But technically, we should not hire him. If something happens and they look at his background check, we will be blamed. I will meet with him and let him know that he can't work here. We cannot risk it."

Just then, we were interrupted by something. I can't remember what it was, maybe a fire alarm, but Andy left before I could respond to what he had just said about letting Jay go.

A couple of hours passed as we both worked frantically, addressing issues left and right. Around 3:15 p.m., I saw Jay waiting to speak to Andy. I started looking for Andy to talk about the situation but was distracted again. Finally, I caught up with him at 4:15 p.m. "So, did you meet with Jay?" I asked.

"No, he is still waiting for me."

"Maybe we should reconsider letting him go. He has done fine in orientation," I said. "How are guys like that ever going to turn their lives around unless people like us give them a chance? Let's give him a chance. What do you think?"

"Sure, you are right. He has been doing a great job. Let's give him a chance," said Andy.

Thirty minutes later, Andy came into my office. "That guy was so grateful he cried for 10 minutes in my office," he said. "I had to shut my door so he could compose himself. He was so used to being rejected he was just expecting it. When it didn't happen, he just could not hold back the tears."

I am grateful to be in a position where I can give people chances. A nursing home administrator has many opportunities to make a positive difference in people's lives—and I'm not talking only of the residents.[4]

Day 247—February 12, 2007

Mr. Bell's rights were violated last Friday, and I let it happen, all in the name of trying to increase our census.

It was late in the day, and the admissions coordinator told Andy and me that we could admit two women on Saturday if we could create a female room. We looked at the resident roster and saw that if we moved Mr. Bell to the middle bed of a three-bed room we could create space for two females. I was told that he had agreed to the move, so the poor guy was taken out of the two-bed room he had shared with his wife, who has been hospitalized for over a week.

So we moved him to the middle bed in a three-bed room. I helped move the beds and the resident. That middle bed is a place of no privacy. The middle bed is the closest you can come to feeling homeless without actually being homeless. It's institutionalized homelessness.

Mr. Bell is alert and oriented, but he cannot speak. He communicates by pointing to visual cues on a board provided by the therapist. But when you look into his eyes, you can clearly see that he understands what you are saying to him. I saw a look of bewilderment and sadness in his eyes when we were moving him, and that expression stayed with me all weekend.

I feel terrible, but I let it happen. In fact, I made it happen and helped with the move. What's wrong with me? So what if he agreed. It was wrong. I was wrong.

This job humbles me like no other. I succumbed to the pressure to have a high census and moved Mr. Bell away from his room and into a place of no privacy. On top of that, I diminished his hope of his wife returning from the hospital to the room they were sharing. Sometimes I disappoint myself. It's hard to be strong enough to always make the right decision when you're weighing business goals versus people, financial pressures versus resident rights.

This morning, I learned that our two new female admissions never arrived on Saturday. And I was so happy. I'd been given a chance to right the wrong I had done to Mr. Bell. So, over the protests of the admissions coordinator, I moved Mr. Bell back to his old room, apologizing to him all along the way.

Ethel, one of the CNAs, overheard my apology and saw the look on my face. "I'm glad you did that, Mr. David, because I visited his wife last night and the nurse said that she might be discharged back here today," she said. "Then they can be together again. That's all they want; is to be together."

She added as she was walking away into the elevator, "So you see, Mr. David, everything is going to work out fine. Don't beat yourself up, Mr. David. It'll be okay. You'll see." She smiled at me and the elevator door shut with a slam.

Day 249—February 14, 2006

No one defaced my last message to the individual who was defacing my postings. It's been there for about a week, and no one has touched it. The strength of the community won!

At the community meeting on the evening shift, I spoke about it, quoting from Stephen Covey's book, *The Speed of Trust*, where Covey talks about how many of the most popular religions around the world preach the golden rule.

I started the meeting by saying: "Respect. Civility. The golden rule. Every major religion preaches it."

I then read the following from Covey's book:

The Golden Rule
Christianity: Do unto others as you would have them do unto you.
Islam: No one of you is a believer until he loves for his brother what he loves for himself.
Judaism: What you hate, do not do to anyone.
Hinduism: Do nothing to thy neighbor which thou would not have them do to thee.

Buddhism: Hurt not others with that which pains thyself.

Confucianism: What you do not want done to yourself, do not do to others.

I said, "Civilizations were built by people following the preaching of the golden rule. Civility = civilization. The same holds true here in our small community of compassionate caregivers. Our success depends on our collective ability to consistently demonstrate respect to one another. How we treat each other determines how we will treat the residents."

I went on to say, "Even subtle forms of disrespect, like leaving dirty linen for someone else to pick up or leaving things a mess in the break room, can erode our community. We all must follow the golden rule."

People were listening intently. I paused, letting the silence linger longer than anyone expected. I wanted the feeling in the room to last as long possible.

Finally, I said: "I felt terrible when we saw someone defacing the postings in the back elevator. But I am so proud to say that you were as offended as I was by that blatant act of incivility. And, ultimately, our community won. My last note to the culprit has been hanging there for seven days and no one has defaced it. You see, the golden rule has strength in our community here."

The staff gave a collective nod, their heads going up and down together as if they'd rehearsed it.

After another long pause, I saw it was 10 minutes to 3:00—time to raffle off the gifts and let the morning shift go home.

The raffle is always fun. I rig it by putting names I've chosen ahead of time in the pot used to "randomly" select the winners. Of course, the staff does not know that I rig the raffles. I don't feel bad about rigging the raffles because I see it as an investment in specific people who are doing the right things and deserve to be rewarded for it. I keep track of who wins, so I can be sure to spread the "luck" around and let many people win throughout the year. I want them all to think they are lucky and winners, if just for one day. Part of being lucky is feeling lucky, and I want my hardworking, deserving staff members to believe they are lucky.

Day 268—March 5, 2007

Today, we finally got the new resident beds the new owners had promised us after they took over. They're electric beds that can be easily raised or lowered, which will make transferring in and out of bed much easier for both residents and staff. The new mattresses will help reduce pressure sores too. Being able to lower the beds helps us reduce side rails that can act as a restraint. This is great. It's excellent. I can hardly believe it.

By keeping their word and investing so much money in equipment that will improve care, the new company has shown staff, residents, and family members that we are on the way up. Now we're on equal footing with other facilities in this region. The new company showed that they care.

Moving new beds in and old beds out was no easy task. But the residents were just fine with the inconvenience in exchange for a new bed. The staff were excited too, as people came to realize that the new beds were high quality and would make life better for us all.

Equipment matters . . . it matters a lot.

Day 275—March 12, 2007

The data paint a beautiful story of the transformation we are witnessing.

Our combined (admitted and acquired) pressure ulcer rate is at an all-time low. We are keeping the number of resident falls and physical restraints down.

The word must be getting out that we're improving things too, because we are caring for more residents than we ever have in the past six years. We have gone from an average of 104 residents a day to 121. We set a record high for occupancy in February, and March is on track to break that record. In fact, in five of the past six months we have set a new five-year high for occupancy. This morning we were 97% occupied. These numbers are unprecedented here—and in most nursing homes in this market these days.

What's more, we are admitting more residents whose stays are paid for by Medicare, averaging 25 now, where we used to average 11. It's all helping to boost our bottom line. We're all proud of the impressive numbers.

We continue to maintain our stellar 29% staff turnover rate, and on many days, when I walk in, I find that all 51 of the scheduled nursing staff have arrived, on time, as scheduled with name tags and smiles on. That's stability—and stability is the key to so much of what really matters to people in long-term care.

We have created the climate that is bringing out the best in our staff. As a result, good relationships are forming everywhere here. Quality of life, human resource outcomes, and clinical care are all improving because the foundation for quality is now in place . . . every day . . . every shift . . . in every neighborhood.

Day 282—March 19, 2007

We added more CNA hours to the schedule. Our occupancy has jumped up so much we were under budget for nursing hours—running under budget in nursing hours is a sin.

When you're adding staff, it's always hard to decide whether to simply add another person to a shift and lower your CNA-to-resident ratios, or to add a "floater" who can serve as an extra pair of hands as needed. Our staffing and relationships are so solid now that we decided that the floater can effectively pitch in and assist where it's needed. Having that extra pair of hands at mealtime and during some of the other peak times can really help.

We added a new floater shift from noon to 8 p.m. This allows one additional CNA to float over two critical meal periods. She can cover other CNAs' meal breaks, welcome new admissions, assist in the dining room, and be that extra set of hands we all need at mealtime occasionally. She's the stress buster.

We have just the right person to fill that slot. And that's the key. Oleni works hard, will not play favorites, and smiles a lot. She has also worked both shifts across two neighborhoods, so she knows all the residents. We are pilot testing this new position with her now. In the next few days, we will meet with Oleni to hear how she thinks the job or tasks or times should be adjusted in order to give the best possible care. If she rises to this challenge, it could really make a positive difference for a lot of people here.

Day 289—March 26, 2007

About a week ago, I got a very disturbing visit from one of our residents. Jenny is about 55 and suffering from cancer and the side effects of chemotherapy. Despite major improvements in our food services, she can't stand our food, so she orders out a lot from the local restaurants, keeping her leftovers in a refrigerator in the nurses' medication room. She tells me it's her taste buds and the effect of her chemotherapy that turn her off to our food.

She was crying when she came to see me today. She said that one of our day shift CNAs, Eric, had eaten her leftover spaghetti. Worse yet, she said, "He's gloating about it and laughing at me."

I was dumbfounded. It was the last thing I expected to hear on a quiet Saturday morning. I said I would speak to Eric and investigate, but she didn't appear to like the sound of that. She was still sobbing when she left my office. I felt lousy, and angry at Eric.

I immediately addressed Eric. When I got confirmation of his actions, I sent him home. He won't work another shift here.

I had an idea. Around 1:00 p.m., I went out and picked up a little refrigerator at Home Depot for Jenny to keep in her room. This way, she can keep her leftovers near her and have access to them when she is hungry. No more minimizing her access and causing her stress.

When I brought it in, Jenny was ecstatic. Later, she wrote me a wonderful, heartfelt thank-you note, saying that I had exceeded her expectations. It felt good to know that I'd been able to hear her concern and come up with a solution that met her needs.

Day 292—March 29, 2007

Today, I presented the following at our quality improvement meeting. This will be my last quality improvement meeting here, so it felt good to be able to give this report:

Accomplishments: June 2006–March 2007

Quality of Work Life Key Measures

- Annualized nursing staff turnover rate over the past 10 months is 28%, down from 77% over the previous 12 months (July 2005–June 2006).
  - The CNA turnover rate has declined from 94% to 38%.
  - The licensed nursing staff turnover rate declined from 43% to 11%.
- We had eight full-time vacant positions in the nursing department on June 12, 2006. By August 15, they were all filled. On September 1, 2006, we established a waiting list of CNAs who want to work here.
- The nursing department's overtime hours declined from an average of 1,400 a month from March through May 2006 to an average of 450 from September through December 2006. Overtime is now a mere 3.6% of payroll.
- The nursing staff has worked short staffed on just 10 occasions in the past 280 days. In other words, there is a less than 3% chance that a neighborhood will work understaffed on any given day.
- Call-offs from nursing department staff, which totaled 52 in April 2006, have declined by 40% over the past 6 months.

Key Clinical Measures

The following quality indicators improved significantly from the first half of 2006 (January through June) to the second (July through December):

- The percentage of residents taking nine or more medications dropped from 58% to 48%.
- The percentage of residents using catheters declined from 8% to 6.5%.
- The percentage of residents who were incontinent and did not have a toileting plan dropped from 9.5% to 0%.
- The percentage of residents whose ability to perform basic activities declined from 11% to 5%.
- The percentage of residents who spend most of their time in bed dropped from 3% to 1%.
- The percentage of residents who are physically restrained declined from 15.5% to 14%.
- The percentage of residents with pressure ulcers who are at high risk of developing pressure ulcers dropped from 25% to 11%.
- The percentage of residents with pressure ulcers who are at low risk of developing pressure ulcers declined from 4.5% to 0%.

Business Measures

- Our average daily occupancy rate has increased from 82% to 94%. We have also increased the number of residents whose care is paid for by

Medicare, which started at 8.5%. Our occupancy and Medicare rates have been increasing steadily as follows:
- June, July, and August 2006 = 107 total and 14.5% Medicare
- September, October, and November 2006 = 114 total and 15% Medicare
- December 2006, January and February 2007 = 117 total and 16% Medicare

- As a result of these changes, our average monthly profit margin increased by 80%. Our profit margin was 15% between November 2005 and May 2006. Over the past three months (December 2006–February 2007), that profit margin increased to 27%.

Day 296—April 2, 2007

Mr. Waitts knows that I'm leaving. I think Celia, one of the CNAs, told him. When he came over to talk to me about it, I told him I'd been presented with a great opportunity to advance my career, but I would miss him.

"Can I still stay here?" he asked. I knew he meant his private room, since he is well aware that I arranged for him to stay there. He also knows that he is poor, with less than $3,000 to his name. I'm not sure whether he understands how his room is paid for. I have explained it to him many times, but he is still fuzzy about MediCal and may think I am letting him stay there for free. No wonder my departure is making him nervous.

"Yes," I said. "I have spoken to the department managers and Andy about you staying in this room. And you can refuse to be moved. That's your right."

I knew I couldn't guarantee anything. He knew it too.

Day 298—April 4, 2007

It's my last day here.

When she said her goodbyes, Kris, the staffing coordinator, told me: "We were not 'just CNAs' to you. That's what made you so different from all the rest of the administrators."

Comments like that make me feel good. One person *can* make a difference. At the same time, I have to remember that the changes we made didn't happen just because of me.

The people who work here make the culture. And there are just a lot of tremendous human beings here. So many caring people here.

So much of what Jim Collins unveiled in *Good to Great* played out here. As he predicted, the problems of commitment, alignment, and managing change largely melted away once we had the right people in place working under the right climate. The right people don't need to be tightly controlled. They do the right thing because they are the right people. They are living angels.

I could have done so much more. I should have done so much more. A lot went right, but I feel that I could have done much more here.

I realize that this is one nursing home in America. I didn't positively change the nursing home world. But I did make some improvements, and I gained tremendous insights into the challenge of trying to change an organization's culture toward person-centered care. It was both a great experience and a terrible one.

I can say that I positively changed Mr. Waitts's world, and he made a positive impact on me. For sure . . . I can say that.

Notes

1. In reading this journal entry now, I see that I need to offer some insight into my motivation for making this move for Mr. Waitts. This was very early in my tenure, and I was still in a research frame of mind, seeing everything in this nursing home world as if for the first time and thinking about the impact physical space has on people. In the case of Mr. Waitts, it was playing out in front of me exactly as I had read about in studies and learned from the experts in the field. He had just been diagnosed with diabetes and had received the first insulin shot of his life. His roommates were keeping him up all night, and he was starting to realize that this was going to be his home. He was poor and had no living relatives. I saw how easy it would be for him to spiral into a depression, and how much having his own room would lift his spirits. I can also see that it probably wasn't fair to others that I provided him with the best room in the facility, and that this act is not something many of my readers will be able to replicate. It's not even a change I could sustain for long, since the next administrator who came along after I left could easily move Mr. Waitts back to a three-bed room. Despite all that, I'm still glad I offered him the room, because he thrived there. Of course, he also thrived because of my daily visits, my questions about his life, and my attention to his pleasures and comfort, and any administrator can replicate those actions.

2. I never did get to have that conversation with my boss, so I never brought Diego back to work. His not being there had a detrimental effect on morale.

3. We eventually learned that Dolmi had stopped taking her medication for manic depression. We learned this from a friend of hers who visited the facility out of concern. Dolmi disappeared shortly thereafter, and we brought Lisa back to work. Lisa was very grateful to have her job back, even though she lost a few days of work without pay. The DHS investigated the incident and did not offer a deficiency. When the investigator saw Dolmi's name as the accuser, she clearly recognized her. Apparently, it was not the first time Dolmi had made these accusations.

4. Jay turned out to be one of our better performers. He had excellent attendance, and he was always willing to assist the female CNAs with whatever they needed. He was true to his word. He had turned his life around, and we were all glad we had given him a chance.

## CHAPTER 1

Leadership

What You Do Matters

Your leadership matters. Quite often people in formal leadership roles are unaware of their impact. Leaders in nursing homes may be more aware of all those you answer to—owners and corporate staff, board of directors, surveyors, families—and not recognize that there are so many people looking to you for guidance and leadership. You have a BIG impact on those who work and live in your building. The role of administrator or director of nursing is a heavy and complex responsibility. Staff, residents, and families seek your intercession daily. Your presence, your responsiveness, and your ability to create a positive work environment directly influence the care your home provides and your organization's overall performance. Because you have such a big impact it is important for you to recognize it and use the influence you have in a manner that promotes a good work environment.

When you have a formal leadership role you work in a fishbowl. Whether you are aware of it or not, you set the tone—people watch what you do. You are modeling the way you want things to go. You can set a tone of teamwork or a tone of "not my job" by how you answer a call bell or walk past it, call housekeeping to clean a spill or pitch in to wipe it up yourself. David Farrell painted the graffiti-covered wall both because he wanted the graffiti removed and because he wanted people to see him doing physical work—work that was "not his job." By stepping outside his traditional role he was actively demonstrating a spirit of going the extra mile. Another administrator assisted the maintenance staff in getting ice from the basement to the dining room when they had special events that required extra ice. The basement did not have elevator access, making this a difficult job. He did it to help, but the impact it had on his staff was far-reaching. Everyone in his building was aware of his stepping in and helping do a job that everyone hated doing. By stepping in in this way he showed his staff that he was not above doing this job. Another administrator had certification as a nursing assistant, and she used it, stepping in when needed. Every snow day, there she was, working alongside the certified nursing assistants (CNAs) on her staff, showing that she was not above doing personal care. By stepping outside of the regular work and assisting staff, leaders demonstrate in a powerful way that they're not too good for the day-to-day work, and that it is not someone else's job—it is everyone's job. This way of stepping in builds teamwork into the fabric of the culture.

You can also inadvertently set the tone in a direction that you do not want. Because what you do is so highly scrutinized by your staff, little things matter a lot. If you hang out with the smokers, because you smoke, other people on the staff may feel left out of an assumed clique. One new administrator said good morning by name to the people whose names she knew, learning later that others, who didn't get their hello by name, felt slighted. These *micro-inequities* are easily remedied, once you are aware of the fact that people watch what you do, take their cues from you, and respond to how you interact with them.

Because you do have a powerful impact it is important no matter where you are in your own leadership development to be aware of your impact and to take deliberate action to use it to model and promote the kinds of behaviors you want to nurture in your building. Sometimes people who are in formal leadership positions are so inundated with all of the day-to-day requirements of their job that they become removed from the primary work that is going on. The enormity of the responsibility has led some administrators and directors of nursing (DONs) to hunker down and get through each day's challenges without taking a step back and looking at how work can flow better and care can be provided better. In this mode you almost stop noticing what is so normal to you, but it certainly isn't the only way, and it may not be the best way, to operate. After all, many of these norms stem from inherited systems that are very difficult to change. In the face of obstacles to change, and the many challenges of day-to-day operations, it is easy to feel powerless to the point of just allowing the status quo to continue even when it isn't working. Eaton described a *vicious cycle* in which current operations create so many difficulties that they absorb all the available time and energy. This sense of inertia happens when leaders see only what they can't change instead of tuning in to the areas where change can happen. If this is what you are feeling, then this book is a wake-up call. You can do something different, and when you do, the results will not only break the vicious cycle, they will also give you momentum for more positive change. You do have an impact. As an administrator or director of nursing you can use your impact daily to create an environment where staff and residents prosper. If you are working in this field and doing all you can to make a difference, then it is our hope that this book will give you both positive reinforcement and some new tools to take on the challenge.

There is something about the organizational makeup of these fragile ecosystems we call nursing homes that makes them very susceptible to poor leadership practices. However, because of their fragility, they are also very responsive to excellent leadership actions. There is a growing body of research-based evidence that leaders of successful nursing homes consistently engage in certain activities that are directly linked to better clinical and organizational outcomes. A leader's actions influence an organization's culture, staff relationships and stress levels, and residents' clinical outcomes and quality of life. In this chapter we walk through some ways of really tuning in and seeing your nursing home from a fresh perspective, and we provide tools to help you generate positive action.

One way to stay in touch with the work and revitalize your own sense of mission about this work is to intentionally mentor staff throughout your building. Being a mentor goes hand in hand with good leadership because good leaders cultivate the leadership abilities of those around them. The basis of good management and supervision is good mentoring relationships. Identify what your employees need to meet high expectations and help them develop their own potential. Tune in to people individually—recognize what they are capable of and what they need to be able to succeed. You will help your managers and supervisors perform better, and you will be a role model for them in their own approach to the people they supervise. This becomes what Eaton describes as a *positive chain of leadership*. By assessing what people need to succeed and then providing the needed support and guidance, you are exercising good leadership in your building.

One administrator realized when he was putting his disaster plan in place that the third-shift nurse supervisor would be the "incident commander" if a disaster occurred during the night. He recognized that he needed to provide the same level of skill development to third-shift staff as to the first and second shifts. He began working regularly with her, during her regular nighttime working hours, to develop her leadership skills. Watching her grow in confidence and ability was, he said, one of the most rewarding aspects of his job. Mentoring staff extends your reach as a leader because you develop that positive chain of leadership that lets you, and staff, know you all can count on good leadership on every shift, whether or not you're in the building.

A big part of people development is setting the tone for and creating an environment that supports and develops *critical thinking*. The culture in long-term care often seems to be the antithesis of critical thinking. As a highly regulated field, there are policies and procedures for almost every aspect of the work. Yet so little actually happens according to plan—most human events have unpredictable elements to them. Because policies and procedures are guides at best, staff always have to think through how to respond to real situations. Furthermore, there are many aspects of the way care is delivered in most nursing homes that do not make a lot of sense. If the long-term care system were to be designed based on what we know today about good practices, it would likely look very different from our current system. Critical thinking, by definition, involves the questioning of our own assumptions and looking for better ways. Fortunately our whole system is undergoing a period of reevaluation and redesign as many established norms are being rethought and new practices are coming to the fore.

To encourage critical thinking we have to be ready, open, and supportive of new ideas and new ways of thinking about the way we work. This can be hard. It is natural to be comfortable with "the way things are," even when we struggle with the difficulties created by our current ways of working. As a leader, when you can engender critical thinking you support staff to find better ways to carry out simple everyday aspects of their work. Rather than bearing with daily stresses, staff can identify points of stress and struggle, and they can brainstorm together how to address them. Administrators and staff who successfully sheltered hundreds of residents in the aftermath of Hurricane Katrina talked about ways the staff came to think analytically and "let their minds go" to come up with creative solutions to overwhelming challenges. In reflecting on the experience, they saw this as critical to their survival and a practice they continued even after the disaster abated.

We have to "create a climate where the truth can be heard," as Jim Collins says. Your openness to everyone's input creates that climate. Sometimes staff concerns can be misunderstood as negativity, when they are actually exercising critical thinking. Take their perspective seriously. If you mislabel staff concerns as "resistance," you may miss the expertise they bring, in knowing what must be addressed for a new practice to succeed. It behooves you to understand what people are thinking. Get to the bottom of staff concerns through dialogue. How you take on a problem matters. If staff trust that their viewpoints will be considered in the process of making changes, they will bring their best thinking forward and offer both their red flags and their ideas for how to address the issues.

In many organizations there is a tendency to gloss over red flags that warn us something isn't working. Collins, in *Good to Great*, notes that the most effective leaders in the companies that made the leap from good to great paid attention to these red flags as early indicators of something amiss and were able to get ahead of the curve to make adjustments before these areas derailed progress. People will only come forward with their red flags if they trust they will be heard. Effective quality improvement depends on this "ground-up" decision making, where the people closest to the situation have the greatest role in identifying problems and shaping solutions. The best leaders facilitate this ground-up problem solving by developing their staff's abilities to think critically. John Maxwell found that *the greatest potential for growth of a company is growth of its people*. People development—mentoring staff at all levels of the organization to develop their critical thinking and collaborative problem-solving skills—is the most effective means of catching red flags early, implementing positive changes, and progressively improving your organization's performance.

Eaton, in "What a difference management makes!", noted that leaders in the low-turnover homes developed leadership at every level of the organization—among supervisors, managers, and peers. This positive chain of leadership is built on staff's intrinsic motivation—what most people who work in long-term care describe as a "calling" to care for others. This intrinsic motivation drives people to overcome the difficulties and stresses of the work to take care of the residents they know are depending on them. When you manage in a way that encourages and supports this motivation, staff step up to the expectation and do their best. When you bring staff into decision making to shape the environment they work in, you help them do their best. One administrator, who took the job at a troubled home, told us one of her first steps was to create work groups to tackle the home's most serious problems, and to enlist participation from all levels of staff in these groups. The home quickly turned around as staff stepped up to the opportunity to contribute to a better environment for residents. She said that including staff in these decision-making and quality-improvement processes made a big difference in turning around staff morale and resident care.

In their research on leadership, Kouzes and Posner found that most people step up to their own personal best when they know that there is an expectation of high standards. It is hardwired into our human nature to want to excel. By having high expectations, leaders tap into a basic human desire for mastery. When management believes staff want to do a good job and provides support, this generates an environment of mutual support. Positive attitudes create a positive environment. In *Encouraging the Heart*, Kouzes and Posner outline these steps for bringing out the best in staff:

- Set clear standards—people need to know what's expected of them.

- Expect the best—it will be a self-fulfilling prophecy.

- Pay attention—tune in to people individually.

- Personalize recognition—group appreciation is good; specific individual acknowledgment is better.

- Tell it in stories—share successes; this is a way of teaching what you're aiming for and acknowledging when you achieve it.

- Celebrate together—have fun; spend at least as much time acknowledging what's gone well as is spent correcting what hasn't.

- Set the example—leaders go first; staff learn far more by what you do than what you say. Model the way.

Modeling the way is the basis for having credibility. Kouzes and Posner refer to it as DWYSYWD, or do what you say you will do. In long-term care this can become an issue, not because of individuals deliberately not doing what they said they were going to do, but because of the fast pace of the work. Too often the action that was taken was never conveyed back to the person who brought up the request, and so that person never hears that the situation has been taken care of. Not closing the loop by getting back to people leaves them hanging, not knowing where things stand, or worse, thinking that you have not followed through. Sometimes you may intend to follow through but lose track because so many demands come your way. It is important to be rigorous in keeping track of areas to be addressed and progress made. It is equally important to communicate the progress to staff so they know you are doing what you said you would do. When you have credibility staff will take your leadership seriously.

In his book *Good to Great*, Jim Collins set out to ignore leadership as a factor in looking at companies that made the leap from being good to being great. His research team was given explicit direction to downplay the role of leadership so as to avoid the simplistic "credit or blame the leader" thinking that is common today. However, what they found was that all of the good-to-great companies had high-quality leadership—traits they called "Level 5 leadership"—at the time of the transition from good to great. Furthermore, the absence of these Level 5 leadership traits showed up as a consistent pattern in the comparison companies that stagnated. His team found that Level 5 leaders built enduring greatness through a paradoxical blend of personal humility and professional will. They were a study in duality: modest and willful, humble and fearless. Other words he used to describe them are not words we commonly use when thinking about or describing great leaders: quiet, reserved, shy, mild mannered, self-effacing, understated, and gracious. But he also found they were fanatically driven and seemed to be infected with an incurable need to produce results. Level 5 leaders channel their ego needs *from* themselves and *into* the larger goal of building a great company. It is not that Level 5 leaders have no ego or self-interest. Indeed they are incredibly ambitious—*but their ambition is first and foremost for the institution, not themselves*. They build strong teams and provide them with the support to succeed.

Good leaders in long-term care have this same kind of passion and drive. At Birchwood Terrace in Burlington, Vermont, Scott West helped his managers build their own teams and develop their leadership skills by teaching them how to hire for their departments. The case study in Chapter 5 describes how he systematically taught them what they needed to succeed, and let them know he had higher expectations for them. He saw his job as a people developer, and his managers grew in their skills as leaders.

Good leaders cultivate and develop the leadership skills of others. In very practical terms this means paying attention to the leadership skills of others and giving people the skill development opportunities they need to become better leaders. For supervisors to lead well, management needs to spend time developing their leadership skills. This can be done through individual coaching and regular peer group meetings focused on supervisory issues. Involving supervisors in workgroups on clinical issues or special projects also creates opportunities for them to develop their leadership skills. Actively involve managers in supporting their supervisors. To begin this work, first assess your managers and supervisors individually and figure out how to help them be their best. See the potential in each and help them develop their potential. It is good to set a high bar. Most people will step up to high expectations. To really develop your people you have to help supervisors and managers take on challenges and grow.

One way to support your managers in their growth is to help them develop trust in their own decision-making abilities. When supervisors ask you to make a decision, use this as an opportunity to help them develop. Help the supervisor think through how to approach the situation, and follow up with them on what happened. One administrator described it this way: First she would tell the supervisor what she saw as the options. They would then discuss the advantages and pitfalls of each option. She would ask for the supervisor's perceptions and share her own throughout the discussion. This thinking out loud, and sharing what you see and how you are thinking about a given situation, gives the other person guidance in the thought process of decision making. Over time, this administrator would start by asking the staff member to list the options, instead of sharing her own perceptions. She would ask the person to list the advantages and disadvantages of each option. They would spend time discussing how each option would play out. This shared thinking and problem solving helps people develop the skill of executive decision making.

Being transparent and direct is essential as you develop people. It is important as you are thinking out loud to spell out the permissions and parameters of the situation so that they can be factored into the staff member's decision-making process. If this important step is glossed over, you may leave people frustrated because they put effort into something without knowing essential information about what could and couldn't be done, and they end up with something that you're not comfortable having them do. When you have concerns about their thought process, spell out the concerns. Enlist their thinking in resolving the concerns. As your staff get more comfortable in taking on decision making, you will also have more confidence in the decisions they are making and be able to support them.

Eventually, they will be making the decisions by themselves; rather than coming to ask for help, they will be coming to let you know what was done in a given situation. You will be comfortable with this because you had a hand in developing the line of thinking that went into the person's decision-making process. In turn, the staff member will be comfortable for having known the parameters and how to think it all through. The person will be able to spell out to you the reasoning that was used, and, even if the path is not what you would have chosen, you will know that he or she figured out a way forward that will work. Keep the dialogue going as decision making is a work in progress.

As you begin the process of people development, it is important to let people know that you are there to support them, and that you are not leaving them out on a limb. It is important to follow up with people because most decisions need continued attention and adjustment. When you follow up with them, you teach them how to follow up and tweak. This continual follow-up and adjustment is another skill for effective management.

You may think it is easier just to do it yourself, but in the long run it is better to grow your staff's ability to make many decisions themselves. The administrator who turned around the severely troubled facility found that as her managers felt competent and trusted, her job as administrator became easier. It was well worth the time she invested in developing them. You may pride yourself in your ability to make good decisions. There's even more pride to be had in fostering good decision makers all around you.

Good leaders always have their eye toward developing the leadership abilities of others on staff. By walking through all parts of your building regularly you will be aware of those staff members who may play informal leadership roles without having formal leadership positions. Tap into their natural leadership by giving them formal leadership roles. Your home will benefit as you involve them. For instance, when you are out and around, you'll see staff who people naturally turn to, talk to, share with, and in general check things out with. They're the ones people always turn to for a hand or guidance, and they're always looking out for others. We call them the "steady Eddies." As you are trying to put in a new practice and form a new committee, you would definitely want to pull them in. Many of these people might be overlooked because they don't speak up in a formal setting or they aren't the loudest voices in a discussion. They may not volunteer for things. You tend to notice more the staff who always step forward and the ones who frequently need correction. You have an untapped supply of reliable conscientious staff who can be developed into shining stars if you notice them and give them the chance. You will also note opportunities for growth and development. For instance, the housekeeping staff member who is so good with residents may be tapped to take the CNA course, or if she doesn't want to be a CNA, she may be a good contributor in other ways—as a committee member, a mentor. Sometimes we forget or don't realize that an opportunity to serve on committees or to be involved in something that's going on has an intrinsic reward for people. By tapping them to be involved, you're telling them that you see them, and you know that they are positive contributors.

This way of being out there in regular rounds each day will also connect you to your staff in a more personal way. You will come to really know and understand their circumstances. You will also know when your staff have needs that you can help with. For instance in one home the administrator heard how some of the staff were having a hard time buying new winter coats. Coats are expensive, and children grow so fast that the coats may only fit for one year. This administrator saw the need and suggested that the home start a coat exchange program. Other homes have given no-interest loans, recognizing that their employees often make so little that credit is not available to them. These loans are typically for car repair or home downpayments. Most report that employees are very appreciative and pay back the loan as soon as possible. Still other homes have instituted food pantries, given flu shots, provided employee lunches or take-home dinners for $4.00 using leftover food from lunch, or provided health clinics for employees and their families who don't have adequate health insurance.

A New Orleans administrator said that he always tried to start his day being out there, making rounds; he knew that it made a positive difference. But before Katrina, there were times that he put corporate demands first and did not get out and around. He felt the difference and knew that everything went smoother when he was out and about the first hour of his day. Since Katrina, he doesn't let anything stop his daily rounds. In the immediate months after Katrina the needs were so great that he had to be out making rounds every day in order to make sure that the home had what it needed to run. Even when things settled back to normalcy, he continued to put this activity first. Everything else is on the back burner until this vital activity is done. He no longer sees it as optional—but as essential.

Being out there or making rounds is not checking *up* on your staff. It is checking *in* on them. Making sure that they have what they need to do their job, and spreading positivity. If you're carrying a clipboard at all, it is a clipboard for notes to yourself about what you want to remember to follow up on. If you are just beginning to make this kind of rounds, know that it will take time for your staff to get used to your presence and to be normal with you around. At first they may be unwilling to really share what their needs are for fear of some sort of reprisal, but as they come to realize that you can be a resource to them, they will let you know what they need. As you follow up, and do what you say you will do, they will be more and more forthcoming.

Work in long-term care can be stressful even under the best of circumstances. As a leader you can help your building run smoothly by purposefully and deliberately taking steps to reduce stress. As you walk through the building note the stress points, and be thinking about how to take them in hand. You can really get a lot of traction by seeing and then acting on the stress inducers in your building. You can reduce stress significantly by getting new equipment that is needed, fixing or replacing broken equipment, and having enough supplies on hand. Make sure your budget has a line item for equipment and supplies. Replace what doesn't work and spend to help staff have what they need to do their job. Following are some examples of real stress reducers:

- Making sure that there is enough linen

- Making sure that there are sufficient lifts

- Checking on broken equipment

- Maintaining adequate staffing levels.

Another source of stress can be a co-worker with very poor people skills or a very negative approach to others. Just as it is important to be explicit in developing people, it is important to be explicit in holding people accountable when they are a detriment to the work and care environment. One of the worst things you can do to your good employees is to allow negativity or unreliability to continue unchecked. As hard as it may be to have the conversation with someone who is negatively affecting others, it is such a great relief to the entire work unit when that negativity ceases, either because the person turns around or is let go. When it feels hard to have a direct conversation of this sort, keep in mind the impact for the whole team as well as for the residents, and be comfortable in asserting that good interpersonal skills are at least as important as good clinical skills in caring for residents and working well with others.

To be effective in reducing stress you have to have your finger on the pulse and really know what is going on for your staff. This means being out there and in touch with your staff. It is how you'll know what needs to be addressed, what needs fixing, where the stress points are, and where your staff needs support. By being out there you learn of their needs and are able to proactively support their work. As someone who works in the building every day, it can become easy to overlook or not see trouble spots.

In your walk through the building you will see what needs fixing or what needs buying. For instance, you note that the nurses' station has broken equipment that needs replacement. In another unit, someone's son was involved in an accident, and you want to be sure to ask how he is doing. You will take note of the things you hear about that will give you an opportunity to support your staff and residents. Again, it is checking in on, not checking up on.

In doing these walk-throughs it is very important to know and use people's names. Some of the recent information on brain activity shows that the pleasure center in our brains lights up when we hear our own name. So being in a leadership position and using people's names has a double benefit—it activates pleasure, and it lets people know that the boss sees them. When he first started, Farrell kept index cards to remember people's names and details about their families. He knew that he could not possibly remember everyone, so he made sure he had a way to remind himself who people were. He used the cards not only to remind himself of names, but also to check to see whom he hadn't had a conversation with recently so he could make sure to zero in on each person individually.

Use this time as an opportunity to pass on the positive. Farrell uses an example of asking a nurse what went well today and having the nurse say how good the lunch was. Further into his walk he puts his head in the kitchen and tells them that the nurse said the residents loved the lunch—"good work guys!" This is an especially good practice when you are crossing departments or shifts that in the busy hectic pace of the work may not be voicing their thanks and appreciation of each other. This is a good time to tune into how things look.

When you're out there on a regular basis, supplies no longer seem to be an issue for people because you note that the CNAs can't find linen and you make sure that it gets ordered—or you troubleshoot the issue between the unit and laundry. You'll note the need for another lift. People will tell you what they need when they are used to seeing you and trust that you will follow through. It is very different for you to come to them than to say my door is always open and expect them to come to you.

It is far easier to do this kind of checking in for your first shift than for your third shift. However, it is important to make the effort on a regular basis for third shift. Third-shift workers often feel overlooked and are quite frequently asked to come to events, trainings, and meetings during time that is their usual sleep time. They resent it when people think that their shift is easy and that all they're doing is watching people sleep. By spending time with them during their work time, regularly, you will be supporting them and informing yourself of the important work that they do. Often third shift has its own culture and approach—people tend to work well together because they have to. Yet they often feel disconnected from the rest of the nursing home life. The quality of work and teamwork on the third shift affects relationships across shifts. So much of the way a day starts depends on how the third shift ends.

When you are trying to focus attention in a special area—whether it be clinical, such as pressure ulcers, or culture change or retention—spending time directly with third-shift staff is more effective than asking them to come to meetings during the day. You can walk through with them what their ideas and issues are in a different way when you are in their milieu. Asking night staff to come to a meeting during the day leaves out your ability to walk through with them, on their terms, what they will be facing and how to handle it. Whether you need your night shift to feel confident in an emergency or you want residents to get a good night's sleep or wake up by their own timing in the morning, being on the night shift with your staff "talking it through" will give you the best information, and them the best opportunity to figure out what they can do to support those goals.

Good leaders share information with their staff. Your organization benefits when you share as much information as you can. This includes financial information. When staff know about the financial situation you are in they can be in it with you in a more informed way. Many homes hold financial information close to the top level of administration. However, David Farrell let his staff follow the data along with him, and they all celebrated their achievements. There's a real benefit to sharing as much information about the financial situation as possible. The more people feel informed about what is going on, the more they have ownership and feel closely connected in a bigger way than just providing care. Everyone who works in the building knows when the census is down. But what they don't know is the specific impact this has on daily resources and therefore daily life. Spelling it out allows staff to be a part of the overall big picture. The financial outlook can be discussed at regular community meetings. Our culture has an almost taboo sense of talking about money and what it means. Leaders may feel *it is none of staff's business. I'm in charge of this; it's my job.* But this way of thinking shuts out the ownership of the work that you are working to encourage.

By opening the channels of discussion about it, you allow people to have a bigger and deeper understanding of the business aspects of providing care. This is not to say that you should ask people to help you make decisions about the budget, but you would do well to tell people how they're being affected by the budget, with enough detail that they can see their stake. For example, coding for the care actually provided can increase revenue. When you begin this kind of sharing, staff can see the positive in taking the extra time to be sure coding is correct. When you don't do this, staff may see their coding corrected without knowing the financial implications, and they may feel micromanaged. When they understand that they are eligible for higher reimbursement because they are already doing the work, but they are not capturing that reimbursement because they are not coding it, and that loss of revenue is added up for them, they can see what a difference their actions can make. If you are thinking about making changes in food service to accommodate residents' preferences, you can let the staff know what is being spent now on food for the residents in their care, and as they think about ways to make changes, they can do so within that budget. Giving people this kind of information treats them as participants in making operations work well for them and for the residents.

Sharing clinical information is a tool for quality improvement. This kind of sharing is really unit-based quality improvement (QI).

A good example is sharing with the staff on the unit that there has been an increase of facility-acquired pressure ulcers. This targeted approach allows the staff to collectively tackle this problem. When they see the quality data for their area of responsibility, collectively, everybody is able to focus on those residents who have the pressure ulcers, for example, and they can figure out together what approaches will work best to heal them and prevent them. This sharing of the data is a good way to open conversations on topics that are timely. How you do it determines how effective it will be. If you merely show the numbers to report problems and exert pressure, people will feel blamed, not empowered. On the other hand, if you show the numbers and have a thorough discussion with the staff about each actual resident that the numbers represent, and figure out with them what can be done, you will have a better chance of turning the situation around.

Making changes often requires having a better understanding of how things are working now. Sometimes when we have worked for a long time in a building, we stop seeing what it really looks like or we don't even notice routines that impede our progress. We walk by things without really seeing them. Many leaders walk past shower rooms without noticing how they are a repository for storage and broken equipment. One nursing home we were working with wanted to convert its bathing areas into "spas." When we all sat down with the CNAs, nurses, and housekeepers on the unit, they rolled their eyes at the thought of a spa. They said, how about fixing the leaks in the tubs so we don't have to manage a wet floor when we are helping residents in and out of the tub. They pointed to the door that is situated in a way that made it difficult to navigate around the room, and the lack of basic space for the residents' belongings. The home's leadership hadn't noticed. When the leaders fixed the leaks and adjusted the door, staff began to trust management's sincerity about making improvements.

As a leader, people count on you to make sure they have a well-functioning, well-maintained physical environment. Farrell paid close attention to the way things looked, and he reaped the benefits of having paid attention. When Farrell painted the graffiti he was not only showing a team spirit by stepping outside of his traditional job, he was also paying attention to the physical environment. When we look at the physical environment there are several areas that are easy to get some traction with and are often not tuned into. We refer to these high-impact, easy-to-address areas as "easy wins." The first is the employee break room, and the second area is the space around the time clock.

These are usually areas that are highly used, primarily by employees, and can, over time, become worn and dingy. Cleaning them up and making them inviting will boost employee morale. For the break room, a coat of paint, some comfortable seating, good food appliances such as working microwaves, and refrigeration will mean a lot to people. As for the time clock, you will want to take note of the kind of signage around it. Some time clock signage may have been put up years ago and never removed. Other signage may be giving a message that you don't trust your staff. You will want to look over the signs carefully and think about what messages you really want to be sending employees. The messages here can be a slight, or a boost, to staff.

Eaton noted the impact of the physical environment on staff. Low turnover homes had a cared-for look to them. When staff know attention is being paid to the physical environment, they respond in kind, also taking extra care of and pride in their environment. Resources to "design on a dime" are available through the Pioneer Network that can help you think about your space and how to make it pleasant to live and work in. Attending to the work and living environment extends beyond the physical appearance, to furnishings and equipment. If equipment is broken, either have it fixed or replaced. Farrell's nurses appreciated his replacing nonfunctional chairs—he demonstrated that he cared about having a reasonably comfortable, safe environment for them to work in.

People take natural pride in a workplace that looks good and functions well. A long-ago study about urban neighborhoods noted that when areas were left overgrown and strewn with garbage, they became more so, and when areas were cleaned up, they often remained cleaned up. When trash is already there, one more piece doesn't seem to make a difference, and when an area is well maintained, it isn't an area for trash to be left in. Making sure staff have well functioning equipment and a nice looking physical environment lets them know you care about their work environment, and you care about them. My InnerView, the country's largest database on staff satisfaction, noted that when staff feel management cares about them, staff is more likely to recommend their workplace to others. A well-cared-for environment indicates a well-cared-about workplace, one with high standards.

When leaders are looking to make changes, sometimes they walk through with new eyes, noting how the building would look to a newcomer. When you're out and about doing rounds or meeting with staff in their work area, take some opportunities to see your building as if you were seeing it for the first time. For instance, that little corner that is not being used—could it be a good place for a coffee pot and a few chairs so residents could sit together and visit? Could it become a cozy corner for residents to take a visitor, for families to sit, or for staff to take a break? Taking pictures helps. A camera can help you see things in a new way. It is easy to take pictures, then put them on an LCD and see the large, sharp images of your building. One home saw through pictures that its residents were lined up in a hallway, slumped over with boredom on a spring afternoon, while the outside patio was unused. It spurred them to make the patio a more comfortable sitting area and bring their residents out into the sunlight. This tool is often used effectively by consultants who come in with new eyes. It works whenever it is done intentionally to take a fresh look at the environment. You'll be surprised at what jumps out at you when you take the time to look. Making changes in the environment that make it easier for staff to do their job well shows them that you care about them.

In an environment where people care about each other and the staff feel that the work environment supports them, they have a positive outlook for getting work done. Then staff really do want to go to the staff party or the holiday get-together because they really like each other.

Your presence, your attentiveness, and your caring really do make a difference. When you care about your staff, it ultimately affects your residents. When staff know that you care and are there to help them, it makes them more willing to help each other and to help each other with residents. When you're in it with them, they're in it with each other. You can have that impact—what you do matters!

## PART II

Practices
for
Stability

## CHAPTER 2

Taking Time to Hire Right[*]

Without question, the most dramatic improvements that occurred in my home described in my journal were a result of personnel decisions. I was struck by how the facility changed after we replaced 20 competent workers with poor attitudes with 20 more effective workers with positive attitudes.

Early in my career, I realized the importance of taking the time to hire right. But not until I got to this nursing home was I able to pull together everything I'd learned and make better selections. Not all of our new employees worked out, but overall they were great people, caring and competent. If you've read my journal, you know how well they performed. In many cases, new employees outperformed veteran staff.

(David Farrell)

PEOPLE HAVE A PROFOUND EFFECT on those around them. New employees affect incumbent staff, both in their ability to perform tasks and in their personality. You're not just hiring their hands and their job knowledge; you are hiring whole persons—their character traits, paradigms, behaviors, communication skills, attitudes, and personality. This means administrators need to get personally involved in the selection process, and they need to know just what they're looking for as they build or add to their team.

In *Good to Great*, one of the key attributes Jim Collins found that all good-to-great companies share is taking the time to hire right. In all 11 of the companies he profiled, executives consistently focused on hiring people with both the right skill set and the right character traits.

---

[*] This chapter builds on content originally developed for and contained in the *Staff Stability Toolkit* produced by Quality Partners of Rhode Island, available at www.qualitypartnersri.org.

Nursing home managers often feel that they can't afford to take the time to screen and hire carefully, but the fact is, you can't afford *not* to. We've all been there: the need to fill staff vacancies is so urgent you put aside hesitation about a potential new hire and "just give them a try." Of course, you get lucky now and then, hiring an excellent staff member through this desperate approach. But in the long run, you are much more likely to find outstanding, compassionate, reliable people to hire if you apply the framework of ideas offered in this chapter.

Two prevailing practices in many nursing homes are the desperation-fueled "any warm body" approach and the hands-off "not my job" approach by administrators and directors of nursing (DONs). Both of these approaches open the door to hiring people who should have been screened out, and it doesn't take long for a home with that approach to go downhill. Your best and brightest staff members get frustrated and leave, only to be replaced by people who may have little aptitude for, or interest in, delivering compassionate, competent, person-centered care.

Taking the time to hire right saves you time in the long run, since it is much likelier that the person will work out and stay for awhile. That means you don't have to spend time refilling the position every few months. If you have churning in your new employees, take a look at your hiring and welcoming process. As you bring in people who are a better fit, and give them a good welcome, they will stay. Good new staff make your organization more stable and increase the likelihood that long-time committed employees will stay.

There are several key elements to hiring the right people. You need to start with having a good pool to hire from. Next comes a good screening process, so you'll hire someone who will likely be effective, reliable, pleasant to work with, and loyal to the organization. Finally, you need to help them settle in, providing an excellent orientation and welcoming program so they'll stay.

Target Ads to Attract the Right People

You need to start by attracting people with the right character traits and skill set. Character traits are far more important than skills, as skills can be learned. To attract a wide enough pool of candidates, you have to cast a wide net—and you have to be sure to cast it in the right areas. You don't want to have just a lot of people applying, you want to have a lot of the right people applying.

Target your advertising to the right people by clearly stating the caliber of person you are looking for. Focus on character traits such as engaging with people, working well with others, and being caring, creative, and compassionate.

Write your ad to appeal to the values of the person you want to attract. Good nursing home employees are not in the field for the money; they truly want to make a difference. Gather a group of staff and brainstorm what your nursing home has to offer, asking why they stay employed. Take the time to clearly spell out your selling points as an employer, and the long-term care's selling points as a field of work. Then capture it in an advertisement. In the ad, give details about whatever you do to support your staff's personal growth, reward longevity, or make work rewarding. Highlight any awards or achievements your home has won, since good people want to work in a place known for giving high-quality care. Include quotes from your staff about what they like about working here. Think about including the following:

- List the names of your past 12 employees of the month. Then write: "If you want to work with some of the best people on earth, and be recognized for your talents and contributions, please apply at Sunny Acres Care and Rehabilitation Center."

- Summarize the high scores from your past staff satisfaction survey.

- Describe a few of the key person-centered care practices you employ to improve residents' quality of life.

- Use a quote from a staff member about what a good place your home is to work in.

Include appealing specifics about the position you're hiring for. For example if you are hiring for a 3–11 certified nursing assistant (CNA) on a homey Alzheimer's unit where staff are highly engaged with residents and work well together, say all those things. If you're looking for a nurse, you might mention how nursing homes offer nurses independence, responsibility, the opportunity to use their assessment skills and develop a specialty as gerontological nurses,[1] and the chance to form real relationships with those they care for and work with. Many nurses are surprised to find how much they love this work once they get involved in it.

Once you've written down everything you want to say, review your ad from the point of view of the kind of person you want to reach. Would this appeal to him or her? Does it stand out from all the other nursing home ads out there? Does it make your home sound as if it is constantly looking for people? An ad that covers several positions indicates desperation and instability. Hiring one good employee at a time will save you time and money in the long run.

Be creative in where you advertise too. Newspaper advertisements are expensive and may not reach your target audience. Ask your staff where they would look if they were looking for a job. Don't overlook the small weekly papers, since many people who are looking for work read them. Think about the day your ad runs. Papers get their highest readership on Sunday, but also consider advertising on the day of the week when the newspaper includes coupons. And consider using Craigslist.com or monster.com to advertise a job opening.

Then track the effectiveness of your ads and change them if needed by noting whether you get a lot of calls or walk-in applicants after you place an ad. Are they people with the character traits you want to attract? Ask applicants what drew them to inquire about a job.

Replace Sign-On Bonuses with Refer-a-Friend Bonuses

Do not overlook your good employees as potential resources—word of mouth is a powerful advertisement. A targeted employee refer-a-friend bonus program is a smarter way to spend scarce resources than paying sign-on bonuses to all newly hired staff. In some areas, sign-on bonuses are so common that nursing home managers think they have to offer them to stay competitive, but sign-on bonuses have many negatives and rarely create the stability that employers are striving for. They can also indicate to a selective candidate that you are desperate for help—not a good sign for someone who wants a stable work environment! Instead, include in your ad that while you don't pay sign-on bonuses, you do pay longevity bonuses, because you value commitment and dependability.

Sign-on bonuses reward people merely for accepting employment, although they may leave as soon as the bonus is paid out. They also send a bad message to the full-time staff who may not have received a sign-on bonus when they were hired. If those employees do the math—and many do—they will see that the cumulative amount of their annual 2%

or 3% increase since they started is less than the amount of the sign-on bonus. Some may think, "Geez, if I quit today and got rehired tomorrow, I'd make more than I do now for showing up every day."

On the other hand, offering refer-a-friend bonuses to your good employees has a double benefit: it gives your best people a chance to earn a bonus, and it provides an additional screen, since good employees usually refer other good workers. This type of bonus also indicates to your reliable staff that you are going to hire good people as their co-workers. In the turn-around facility in Farrell's journal, the refer-a-friend program he instituted brought him some excellent employees.

Refer-a-friend programs also increase the likelihood that both the people doing the referring and those referred will stay. In his book *First Break All the Rules*, Marcus Buckingham highlights a Gallup study that found that organizations where staff have a "best friend" at work have lower turnover rates than other organizations. Why? Simple—work is more pleasant when you have friends nearby, and best friends talk each other out of looking for another job.

Farrell tested some hypotheses that made his referral program more effective. He learned that it works better to pay the bonus in full when the new person is hired or immediately after he or she completes orientation. Most nursing homes pay in increments over a period of time (30 days, 90 days, six months, one year), and only pay if the new employee is still there when each deadline is reached. He found the practice of incremental payoff of the bonus highly ineffective, as it makes the staff who referred the friend who was hired feel that their effort was not worth the trouble. In their minds, if you hire someone they referred to you, they completed their part of the equation. If you have a good screening and welcoming process, you'll make a good hiring decision and help a good new employee stay. Paying out the total bonus amount quickly often motivated the employee to refer another friend.

It is important to actively promote the refer-a-friend bonus program to all staff, posting a flyer about the program in the employee break rooms and by the time clock, attaching it to paychecks, and talking up the program at department head and general staff meetings. Farrell took it a step further. To increase the likelihood of attracting the very best candidates, he specifically targeted his top employees individually, asking them to refer people they knew. By focusing on his best staff, he trusted that they would make good referrals. He let them know how much he valued them, and that he trusted their judgment.

To make sure this important task did not get pushed aside by more "urgent" concerns, Farrell created a protocol to follow. First he met with the leadership team, nursing schedules in hand, and identified the top 40% of the nursing staff, considering criteria such as reliability, competency, relational skills such as listening and communication, supervisory skills, and trustworthiness.

Then they divided up the list among the leadership team members. Over the next week, each leader from the meeting met individually with the employees on his or her list, asking them to refer their friends. They met with the top-performing, newest employees first, because they typically had just come from another facility where they likely knew former co-workers who were looking for a better place to work.

Farrell's team told their top performers: "We want to hire other people who are just like you." They then took the time to explain that they were asking all their best workers to recommend other good workers to hire, since they trusted that they had friends with similar good character traits and work ethics. Finally, they said: "We would rather pay our best people for a referral than anyone else."

Farrell kept track of their referrals as job candidates started coming in, paying careful attention to who referred whom. If someone had been referred by a lower-performing staff member, they were extra vigilant during the screening and interview process. They always asked how long the referring employees had known the person they referred and why they had referred that person. If their first answer was, "to get the bonus," the team rarely hired the referred person. But if the employee said, "Because she is an excellent nurse and a really great person," they usually made a good hire.

The process worked remarkably well for Farrell's team.

If your staff is hesitant to refer their friends, ask your reliable employees why. You may have to adjust your organization's culture to ensure better treatment for staff.

Always Be on the Lookout for Talent

Long-term care professionals should never stop recruiting people into the profession, staying alert for the character traits and service attributes that make for an excellent employee wherever they go. Some of Farrell's best hires were people with no previous experience in long-term care, who may never have considered the career if someone had not mentioned it to them as an option:

Early in my career, I recruited some of the best employees from a Burger King near my nursing home. As I sat there eating my lunch or nursing a soft drink, I would carefully observe the Burger King staff to see who smiled, displayed a solid work ethic, and seemed to enjoy serving others. I knew that I had a better job that would mean much more to a people-person than flipping burgers, as long as they were able to complete the CNA class. Those former fast food workers turned out to be some of my best CNAs.

Maintain High Standards and Wait for the Right People

Poor hiring decisions compound stress and instability. Even when staff are tired and urging you to hire to fill vacancies, they want you to take the time to hire reliable, friendly co-workers who care as much as they do. If you do not, they will only end up working even harder—and often while building up resentment. We've all seen frustration on the faces of some of our best people as they train a new worker they know will likely not work out.

On the other hand, each well-chosen new employee infuses the organization with more positive energy as another cheerful, hardworking person joins the staff.

Key steps that make it easier to hire excellent people include the following:

- Create an effective screening process.

- Include a range of staff in the interview process.

- Focus on character traits first, not skills, because skills can be taught while caring cannot.

Enlist Your Receptionist as a Key Member of the Recruitment Team

You only get one chance to make a good first impression. Think about the impression you are making on potential employees, so you get off to a good start with the caring, committed people you want to attract. The first step is making sure your receptionist understands that she plays a key role. Potential employees consider how they were treated by the first person they interacted with when considering you as an employer, and that first contact is often with the receptionist.

Farrell strengthened his receptionist's role in the recruitment and hiring process in a number of ways. First and foremost, he let her know how important she was to their success, talking about the importance of providing job candidates with a good first impression. He also asked her to help assess candidates for their friendliness and communication skills, since she could observe them when they didn't think they were being evaluated. He found he could learn a lot by asking his receptionist about how the individual candidates interacted with the residents and other staff while filling out their application.

If your facility has a recruitment and retention committee, make sure the receptionist is on it. You might even ask the receptionist to serve as the chair, to make sure this person understands his or her critical role and is prepared to put the home's best foot forward.

Another reason to empower the receptionist is that high-quality job seekers are likely to be filling out applications all across town the day they come to your facility. They will appreciate a warm welcome, being offered a cup of coffee and a comfortable place to sit.

Make sure your receptionist

- knows that active recruitment is always happening

- always knows which positions are available and has copies of each job posting

- has applications, pens, and employee benefits information available at the desk

- knows where the applicant should sit (among the residents) to fill out the application

- has a clear plan for notifying a designated person from administration whenever an applicant comes in so that the candidates will be screened right away.

To facilitate that process, you need a designated area at the reception desk with everything needed for new applicants (legible applications, pens, etc.) and a receptionist checklist (see below) for handling applicants. Box 2.1 provides a sample checklist for your receptionist to keep at the front desk.

Box 2.1
When Someone Comes in to Apply for a Job

1. Warmly greet them, and begin assessing how warm and friendly they are. Did they return your warm greeting? Pay attention to their communication skills.

2. Give them an application and a pen.

3. Ask what position they are applying for.

4. Escort them to where they should sit to fill out the application (among the residents).

5. While they are completing the application, notify [add the name/title of the person you want contacted here] that a candidate is available. Tell them what position the person is applying for.

6. Let the candidate know someone will be with them shortly. Point out where the restroom is and offer water, coffee, or tea.

7. Notice whether and how the candidate is interacting with residents or staff.

8. Jot down your first impressions of the candidate and pass the note to the supervisor when you pass on the application. The note may look something like this: "Seems nice. Polite. Good communication skills. He was talking with Mr. Jane. Two of our CNAs—Maria and Carol—seemed to know him."

Screen Every Applicant Yourself

Farrell always instructed his receptionist to page him no matter what he was doing, so he could interview the prospective employee on the spot. He said that nothing was more important to him than getting the right staff on board and making sure his employees weren't working short. You would be wise to interview candidates that walk in, and thereby seize your chance to get to know a good prospective employee before the next employer does, since they won't be on the job market long.

We strongly recommend that the administrator take on the role of screening every applicant, since there is nothing more important to an organization's success than hiring high-quality, compassionate people. By screening each applicant, the administrator can save each department manager a lot of time, since they will need to interview only those candidates that the administrator feels good about. It makes sense for one designated person to play this critical role of screening applicants for their character traits.

> I learned early in my career as an administrator that I couldn't sleep at night when someone that I did not feel good about had just been hired and now worked for us. Screening every applicant myself was the best way to guarantee a good night's sleep.

The process of screening every applicant involves ascertaining whether or not this person is a fit for your organization, tuning in to the character, personality, and behavior traits that affect how—and how well—they relate to other people. In his first meeting with a candidate, Farrell asks the key questions listed in Box 2.2. Rather than write down their answers, he simply asks questions and watches people closely as they answer. At this point in the screening process, he is not that interested in their job history. While he wants to know what type of position they are qualified for and what job they are interested in, beyond those basics, his main focus is on who they are as people. Talking to them in this way lets him know their ability to communicate and their general friendliness.

> I also counted the number of times the candidate smiled while we were together, looking for at least five true smiles. I call this the five-smile rule, and it has helped me pick good people for years. People who naturally smile frequently in their interactions with others are probably friendly, service-oriented people who will lift the spirits of the residents and their co-workers. People who don't smile don't get past my screening process.
>
> A simple way to count the smiles is by marking an "x" under each smiling face on the page where you keep your interview questions and notes. [See Box 2.2.]

If the candidate answers these questions (or the ones you choose to ask) to your satisfaction, walk him or her through the facility so you

Box 2.2
Key Questions Farrell Asks in His Initial Interviews

- Share with me the nicest thing you've ever done for someone. Got any stories to illustrate that you've been compassionate?

- Who is the nicest person you know and why?

- What does trust mean to you?

- Do you always tell the truth?

- What do you do for fun? What activities do you enjoy when you are not working?

- What are you most proud of?

- Tell me about your prior experience(s) in caregiving.

- Where?

- How long were you there?

- What are your feelings about the experience there?

- In what ways were you recognized there?

- What were some challenges that you encountered there?

- Tell me about a time when a resident refused to eat or take a bath. How did you handle it?

- Tell me about a time you had a conflict with a co-worker. What did you do?

- Tell me about a time when you were confronted with a policy that you didn't believe in. How did you handle it?

- Tell me the first names of three elders you had a close relationship/friendship with in your last job? (Note their reaction and speed of remembering the elders' names.)

- Of all the work you have done, where have you been most successful?

- What motivates you?

- Can you provide us with a copy of your last performance review and current attendance record from your last/current place of employment?

can see how the person reacts and interacts with others. Here are some things to be on the lookout for:

- Does the candidate give a warm greeting to everyone he or she passes?

- Does the candidate look people in the eye when greeting and speaking to them?

- Does the candidate appear to enjoy interacting with others?

- Does the candidate exhibit active listening skills?

- Does the candidate appear confident, poised, and relaxed?

Make sure you can observe candidates interacting with residents by setting them up to do so. The first step is having candidates fill out their application in a spot where residents are sitting. The second would take place during the tour.

> I'd make sure the job applicant is standing next to a resident who I know would likely engage with the candidate, and then I'd pretend I had something to do, telling the applicant that I'd be right back. Then I'd walk away and pretend to do something at the nursing station while observing the candidate to see if he or she engaged with the resident. If they inched away or said nothing, I was not impressed, since I wanted to hire people who genuinely like elders and want to talk to them.
>
> I also took note of each staff member we passed when going through the facility with a candidate. After the tour was over, I'd ask the candidate to wait in the lobby while I retraced my steps, asking everyone we had passed if they know or have worked with the candidate. That sometimes yielded valuable information. Your own employees can be the best reference checks you'll ever get.

After Farrell finished with the candidate, he would decide whether the person got a second interview with the appropriate department manager. He used the following tool in Box 2.3, highlighting all the traits that applied.

Box 2.3

Requirements for a Second Interview

Traits Desired	Behaviors Observed
Friendliness	• Smiles with both mouth and eyes • Takes active part in conversation • Actively listens or reflects back other people's words and gestures • Uses humor appropriately • Pleasant tone of voice • Firm handshake • Smiles, greets, and makes eye contact with others
Courtesy	• Lets interviewer finish talking before responding • Uses courteous words ("Please," "Thank you," "Nice meeting you") • Makes appropriate small talk while waiting • Holds doors open, steps aside to let others pass by
Responsiveness	• Uses no long "uh's" before answering • Goes beyond "yes" and "no" answers to questions • Volunteers information without interviewer having to prod for more information • Answers the question asked; does not evade difficult questions
Empathy	Listening behaviors include: • Head nodding when appropriate • Overall slight muscle tension, indicating alertness and energy associated with caring • Slight leaning forward • Eye contact • Paraphrasing to show understanding • Communication of feelings when substance warrants it
Assertiveness	• Asks for what he or she needs in interview (clarification, information, time) • Volunteers pertinent information not asked for • Discloses negative information truthfully • Sounds confident and forthright, both in tone of voice and in words used

Build Ways of Testing Reliability into the Interview Process

For candidates who make it through that first screen, set up two or three mandatory appointments to test reliability. Those appointments should span a very short time period, so as not to drag out the hiring process. For example, the department head might set up a second appointment with the candidate within a few hours of meeting the candidate, asking the person to come back later that day.

Not only can you see if the person is on time for the appointment, but you can learn a lot from the answers provided by a candidate who can't make the appointment. For instance, a candidate may have another full-time job where he'll need to be at that time. Another may say she can't come back at 3 p.m. because she depends on her son to drive her, and he won't be available then. In those cases, you've learned something about potential barriers to availability that you will need to take into consideration.

Scott West, whose story as Birchwood's administrator is captured in the case study in Chapter 5, built three separate appointments into his interview process over a very short period of time. The first visit was an open house and walk-through. The second visit was an interview with the manager for the position being applied for. The third visit was a medical screening. Anyone who couldn't make all three was automatically eliminated. After all, if candidates could not keep three appointments when they want a job, how could he rely on them to show up once they were hired?

Teach Your Department Managers How to Hire Right

Department heads may be hesitant to hire staff, or make poor hiring decisions, because they have never been taught how to do it. Help them learn this skill by teaching them the essentials of hiring (see Box 2.4).

Include Other Staff, Residents, and Family Members

Staff members, residents, and residents' family members can provide important perspectives in evaluating a candidate.

Lori Todd, the administrator at Loomis House, in Holyoke, Massachusetts, includes frontline staff, residents, and family members from

Box 2.4

The Ten Steps to Teaching Department Managers

1. In a department head meeting, explain that managers need to get involved in hiring so they can help make a good selection and can better help new hires settle in.

2. Ask those who have experience in hiring to share tips so the others can learn from their experience.

3. Go over some basic do's and don'ts of what to ask in an interview.

4. Talk about how to review an application, using applications of recent hires who did not work out. Have your managers work in groups of three to look for red flags. Then bring the group back together to discuss what they found.

5. Have them review applications of recent hires who have been employed more than six months and are doing well to look for indicators of success. Talking this through with the group will help managers think about what they need to look for in an employee.

6. Work together to develop interview questions, including some for everyone and some specific to each department. Think about typical situations encountered on the job where an individual's character traits and judgment make a difference, and how to use these as discussion points in an interview.

7. Practice interviews with co-workers, so managers who aren't comfortable doing interviews have some experience and get some feedback.

8. Talk through a game plan for walking a prospective employee through the building. What do you want to look for during a walkthrough? How do you want to provide opportunities to see applicants interact?

9. In future management meetings, check in to see how new hires are doing and discuss how to meet their needs.

10. Spend a little time together reviewing who worked out, who didn't, and why. Then decide whether and how your hiring practices should be revised to lead to more successes. Pay close attention to whether the problem was a bad hiring decision or an insufficient welcoming process.

the neighborhood in the hiring process when a caregiving position is being filled. Since the residents are the ones being cared for, she says, they should have a say in who is hired. Also, residents sometimes pick up on something important about a candidate that staff missed.

Staff involvement provides many benefits. First, it boosts morale by including employees in an important process—though this will work only if you genuinely want and consider their input. Second, when co-workers invest time in interviewing a potential hire, they are more highly invested in that person's success if they join the staff. The interview process also lets people get to know each other a little, so new employees see familiar faces on the staff when they start work, increasing the odds that they will stay. But in addition, when people who actually do the job evaluate a candidate for that job they are more apt to notice potential strengths and weak points in a candidate that a supervisor may not see.

Lori developed a list of questions for the nonmanagers on her hiring teams, so she could be sure they would stay within legal limits. Another benefit of having uniform questions is that asking everyone the same questions makes it easy to compare candidates, along with any new questions that come up during the interview.

To develop her list, Lori gathered people who wanted to be part of the process and asked them to write down the questions they would want to ask a candidate for hire. Her human resources person then modified the questions, preserving their essence while making sure they met legal standards. See their interview questions in Box 2.5.

These questions help interviewers get a feel for the interviewee's critical thinking skills, judgment, and character. Lori finds that this additional screening saves time and money by reducing turnover and it nurtures close relationships between residents and staff and among staff.

Provide Affordable Health Insurance Benefits for Employees

David Farrell observes:

> For a long time now, I've questioned our field's approach to employee health insurance and paid time off. Our stingy approach saves money up front on one line item, but it is one of the main factors contributing to our high turnover rates.[2] I believe it costs more than it saves. The impact on revenue is hard to calculate, but the human costs are clear. Turnover results in errors, low morale, and poor service.

Box 2.5
Loomis House Interview Questions for Residents, Staff, and Family Members

- What do you do when you are stressed?

- Tell us about a stressful situation that happened while working and how you handled it.

- What made you decide to become a CNA (or other position)?

- What do you feel you do very well? (What do you feel are your strengths?)

- What do you feel you would like to do better? (What are your challenges?)

- Can you tell us what you consider to be abusive?

- If you were to witness abuse or had been told by someone about an abusive situation, what would you do?

- What would you bring to Loomis House if you were to be hired?

- What do you expect from Loomis House if you were to be hired?

- What would you do if you were in a situation with a resident where you shouldn't leave, but you are asked by someone in authority to go and handle another situation? (Example: You are the only CNA in the second floor dining room, there are 15 residents in that room, and a nurse asks you to go toilet Mrs. K.)

- If a 96-year-old resident was going toward the door to leave and said to you that she was waiting for her mother to pick her up for lunch, how would you respond?

- If you were going in to care for a resident who was agitated, how would you handle it?

It may sound costly, but I believe that we need to start using the opposite approach to benefits if we are serious about reducing turnover. Instead of offering benefits that only half the staff can afford, or encouraging staff to waive their right to health care coverage for an extra dollar or so an hour, we should offer affordable benefits and encourage all employees who need them to make use of them.

For employees whose spouse provides their health coverage, opting out of an employee's plan in exchange for extra pay is a great option, but this practice has serious consequences for those without spousal coverage. Forced to choose between higher wages and health care, low-wage workers often opt for the higher wage, gambling that their health will remain good because they need extra cash to pay the bills. This puts them—and the residents who depend on them—in a precarious situation and adds a great burden of stress to their lives.

Think how much better it would be for your employees if you offered them all affordable health benefits, perhaps utilizing a sliding scale for premiums based on an employee's rate of pay. When your employees have health insurance, they can take care of their medical needs before they become medical emergencies, and scheduled absences are far less disruptive than unscheduled absences due to emergencies. Your employees will be in better health with better attendance when they have routine access to preventive care and treatment for chronic injuries and illnesses. Furthermore, offering affordable benefits would make your organization a more attractive employer, allowing you to be that much more selective in your hiring practices.

A home in Louisiana that participated in staff stability programs as it recovered from Hurricane Rita, took this recommendation to heart. It made its health insurance benefits affordable for all of its employees, many of whom took up the benefits. A year later, this benefit turned out to be a prime reason for its improved retention. When asked about it, staff said that the benefit was important and so was the fact that the management cared so much about their health and well-being.

Hire for Full-Time Positions, not Piecemeal Part-Time Staff

If you're focused on delivering person-centered care, it stands to reason that you need to examine the composition of your staff. Measure the percentage of full-time staff (the number of full-time staff divided by the total number of staff). If less than 80% of your staff works full time, make some changes to increase that percentage. The higher the percentage of full-time staff, the greater the potential for staff to deeply know the residents and each other. That is why it is so important to hire full-time employees whenever possible, instead of plugging holes in the schedule with part-time staff. Having too many part-time staff also makes the schedule unwieldy for managers to handle, increasing the likelihood that staff will find themselves working short.

Many nursing homes have a high percentage of per diem and part-time staff, especially among their licensed nurses. Residents and full-time staff suffer when there are too many part-time employees, especially among those in supervisory positions. Just look at the problems:

- Per diem nurses may not be there from one day to the next to follow up on clinical issues, receive a return call from a doctor, answer a family member's questions, or pass on key information to other caregivers, such as the reason for requesting a lab test. Staff who are only present part time can't recognize subtle changes in a resident's condition that may be early signs of a more significant problem. If you don't know Mabel's baseline, how do you recognize a change in her condition?

- Per diem and part-time staff can't participate fully in facility-wide quality improvement or culture change efforts. For the most part, they are simply filling a shift, performing tasks to meet the resident's basic needs and keep the facility compliant. Many part-timers are not knowledgeable about or close to the residents, they don't have close working relationships with their co-workers, and they know little if anything about the home's policies and organizational culture.

- Nurses who work part time usually don't take ownership of anything beyond their own shift assignment, so they often don't take the extra time to organize the medication cart, the medication room, the charts, and so forth. Per diem staff often do not feel vested in the organization because they aren't there very often. Often, this is their second job, and they treat it accordingly.

- CNAs do not get stable supervision if their supervising nurses are part time. They may be expected to do things one way on Mondays and another on Wednesdays, and they may not have anyone who knows and appreciates all that they do or who they trust enough to turn to if they have a problem. This lack of consistency and support contributes to CNA turnover.

Certainly there are per diem and part-time staff who are committed to your organization and reliable in their schedule. See if they will convert to full-time status or accept a regular schedule where you can count on them and they are engaged in facility-wide efforts that go beyond the shifts they work.

> I have sometimes gone so far as to create a full-time position for the right person, even if the schedule indicated a need for help just a few days a week. Finding the shifts to offer the candidate a full-time job was usually just a matter of reducing the hours worked by a few lower-performing, unreliable part-timers.
>
> Converting our staff from mostly part time to mostly full time played out beautifully in my turn-around home. The continuity that resulted reduced stress, supported good communication, and built positive momentum. In an organization that had long suffered from chronic instability, people noticed that consistency felt good.

The same thing happened at Birchwood (described in Chapter 5). In June 2005, Birchwood Terrace was having a retention problem. It also had more nurses working per diem or on the Baylor system than it did full time. Birchwood's managers soon realized they were inadvertently creating incentives for people not to work full time by paying more to those who didn't.

They resolved to increase their full-time staff, revamping their bonus system to reward only full- and part-timers who worked guaranteed hours. They stabilized their staffing, and Birchwood soon got a reputation as a good place to work. The change also improved Birchwood's relations with hospitals, medical staff, and families, as people learned they could rely on their continuity. As a result Birchwood had a waiting list of nurses who wanted to work for them—full time.

Give Your New Staff a Good Welcome

Nursing homes in a staffing crisis often try to fill a hole on the floor by hurrying along the orientation of new employees, putting someone to work before the person has had adequate preparation.

The day's shortage may be resolved—at least on paper—but how good is the care that is being provided? And how long will new people stay if they are left floundering, expected to shoulder a full workload before they've gotten to know the residents or the routine? Under this scenario, it is not unusual to see a new employee depart within a few weeks. Some just leave during their break and never come back.

This approach to orientation is especially tough for people new to CNA work, since certification classes do not adequately prepare people for the real-life challenges of the job. But even experienced workers need time to get to know your residents, staff, policies, and values. It is important for new nurses, too, because there is a big difference between learning clinical skills and supervising a shift.

New workers need time to gain confidence, apply their skills, and learn the ropes in the neighborhood or unit where they will be working. This will vary depending on their level of experience, and the complexity of the residents they are caring for.

New employees need to be checked in on frequently during their first days and weeks. The highest rates of turnover for most facilities occur within the first 90 days of employment. Part of the reason is the tendency to hurry through a partial orientation and then leave new people to make it without assistance too soon after they start on the job.

> I personally check in with new employees frequently for their first few months. Usually, I say something like, "Are things still going well for you here?" or "Do you like working here so far?" or "Is everyone who works here treating you well?"

To close the loop, and to be sure that everyone is supporting the new worker, keep your managers and supervisors abreast of where new staff are in this process. Make sure to follow up closely on people hired to work weekends.

Properly welcomed health care professionals are more likely to feel good about the new position, quickly integrate with their co-workers, and stay on the job. They are also quicker to develop a sense of teamwork and a commitment to their new role.

Here are some successful strategies you can adopt as part of your staff orientation:

- Make the first day a celebration. First impressions of the new job are permanent. Avoid extensive lectures, tedious presentations of policies and procedures, and interminable paperwork on the first day. Instead, focus on making the new person feel special and welcomed. Consider welcome signs, team lunches, or a celebration cake. Digital cameras make it easy to post the new person's picture in the staff lounge with a welcome sign below it. During the newcomer's first hour on the job, conduct an enthusiastic tour of your entire facility. Get the new person out among the employees and residents.

- Use adult learning methods—role-plays, multimedia, stories, brief videos, hands-on experiences, demonstrations, and interactive exercises—to convey the information you need to pass on. Spread out your administrative paperwork to several short sessions during the first week.

- Make sure that new employees' work areas, badges, uniforms, paperwork, keys, and entry codes are ready for them on their first day.

- Follow a checklist of the entire orientation process for each new employee, to make sure you don't miss a step for anyone.

- Pay for new staff members' meals during their first week on the job.

- Create multiple opportunities for your new staff to meet with employees from all departments throughout your facility. Introduce new staff to the residents who will be under their care.

- Assign a mentor to new staff to help them learn the ropes and give them someone to turn to if they have a question or encounter a challenge. Train mentors in communication and sensitivity to different ways people learn. Provide mentors with support from their supervisor and a regular avenue for giving progress reports on new employees. Compensate staff for this extra responsibility. Recognize that new employees turn to their mentors long after they have settled in, so make this mentor position a permanent, ongoing role.

- In making up the assignment for a new employee's initial period of employment, consider the optimal circumstances for a success. Put new employees under the wing of a supervisor who is good at developing people. Sometimes new employees are put where there has been a recurring vacancy. This just places another new staff person into an unstable situation and increases the likeli-hood this new employee will also not stay.

- Make sure new staff have a consistent assignment that has the right level of responsibility to match what they can handle as they settle in. One common problem is assigning a new employee to a very challenging group of residents, the assignment that nobody else wants. This places the new person in an unstable situation. Instead, concentrate on creating a stable environment for the ini-tial period of employment to allow new staff to settle in. Give new employees an assignment that will not send them running for the door, and give them the same assignment for at least two months, so they have time to get to know residents and co-workers. If the regular assignment will be weekends or nights, orient on week-days when supervisors and managers are available to provide sup-port. Then shift the new employees to their regular assignment when they are comfortable and confident. Pay attention during the transition to the new assignment.

- Regular oversight by management and supervisors increases the likelihood that a new employee will stay. Have supervisors and managers introduce new staff to their duties, their co-workers, and the residents, and make sure they check in with new employ-ees a few times a day during the first week and daily for the rest of the month.

- Complete paperwork, but spread it out over the first few weeks. Administrative paperwork such as employment agreements, ben-efit packages, and insurance policies should not take up all the time of your new hire orientation. One common mistake is to try to get everything done on the first day.

- Assign meaningful work and hands-on experiences. Rarely will new employees remember everything that is thrown at them dur-ing their first few days on the job. However, they will remember a hands-on experience. For example, have them attend a care confer-ence, observe a meeting, or assist in activities. Meaningful hands-on work makes staff feel more rapidly integrated into their job.

- Schedule short meetings for new employees with all department heads to give them a broad overview of your facility and each department's function. Let them see that everyone is working toward the same goal of excellent person-centered care and service.

• Explain your facility's vision, goals, culture, and accomplishments in a well-designed brief presentation using slides, video, or multimedia.

Effective orientation takes more than a day or two. Some staff need to ramp up slowly to a full workload. For example, a newly certified CNA that was hired will likely fail if given eight residents to care for after just five days of orientation. Instead, try starting the newcomer with four residents, then move up to six and then eight. Letting employees proceed at the pace that is right for them increases their confidence and likelihood of success. You may not feel you have the time for a slow process, especially when staff are working extra hard to make up for a vacancy. However, if a potentially good employee leaves because of being overwhelmed, you have to start all over again. Many people grow well into the work when they have a good process of orientation and welcome.

Keep the Focus on Retention

Too many organizations make the mistake of focusing mainly on recruitment, but constantly recruiting new staff will only create chaos if your nursing home is not able to retain them. As long as you have instability, you'll feel pressure to lower your standards and recruit indiscriminately. But once you've stabilized your staff, the rest will follow.

Ultimately, the best way to stabilize your home is to keep your best staff. Good staff make residents and their family members happy, and their word of mouth will be your best selling point.

So what makes staff stay? In their analysis of more than 100,000 nursing home staff satisfaction surveys, My InnerView found that staff said three things made them stay on the job and recommend their workplace to others:

1. Management cares.

2. Management listens.

3. Management helps with job stress.

In other words, helping your managers become caring, supportive, effective supervisors is the best thing you can do to reduce turnover and create staff stability, thereby reducing your need to hire.

Notes

1. This is a key element in the nationally recognized LEAP (Learn, Empower, Achieve, Produce) program.

2. The American Health Care Association (*Report of Findings—2008 AHCA Nursing Survey, Nursing Staff Vacancy and Turnover in Nursing Facilities*) estimates that CNA turnover averaged 66% a year nationwide in 2007.

## CHAPTER 3

From Absenteeism to Attendance*

LOREN SALVIETTI, ADMINISTRATOR AT Quaboag-on-the-Common in West Brookfield, Massachusetts, found that attendance problems were her leading cause of terminations. She often found that she was letting people go who otherwise were very good employees. Tired of losing these good employees, she decided to do something different.

First, she called other administrators in the area to see if anyone had a policy that was working for them. No one she talked to did. They had policies; they just didn't work. Frustrated with the lack of a model policy that would actually improve attendance, she decided to create her own. So she put together a policy that she thought had the potential to help attendance, then quietly put it in place for one year to pilot test it. After the first year, she held staff meetings to both inform her staff of what had been happening and openly discuss the policy. She

---

* This chapter builds on content originally developed for and contained in the *Staff Stability Toolkit* produced by Quality Partners of Rhode Island, available at www.qualitypartnersri.org.

started her meeting by telling her staff: "You're all adults. I trust that you are responsible. If you can't come to work, I know you must have a good reason. I'd like to work with you so you can take care of important matters in your life and I can still be sure that we can count on you when you're on the schedule."

In these meetings, which were held at different times over a period of several days so all employees could attend, Loren introduced the policy and asked for staff reaction and input. The policy (reproduced at the end of this chapter) was modified based on those staff discussions and then put in place.

By shifting from a punitive policy to a respectful, constructive, helping, flexible policy, Loren reduced terminations due to attendance from 40 in one year to 1 in the next. Daily attendance at her facility improved significantly. Salvietti's attendance policy is exactly the kind of practice that differentiated homes in Susan Eaton's study, "What a difference management makes!" Eaton found that one of the greatest differences between homes with high turnover and homes with low turnover was their approach to employee attendance and scheduling practices. Those homes that treated staff as Loren did had low absenteeism and low turnover.

Understanding Understaffing and the Vicious Cycle of Turnover

David Farrell attributes his success as an administrator to his obsession with preventing understaffed shifts. Understaffed shifts are often the greatest frustration of both nurses and certified nursing assistants (CNAs), both because of the increased stress for staff and because of the negative impact on care. So Farrell focused on making sure to be fully staffed on every neighborhood, every shift, every day. His focus and actions greatly reduced the staff's stress level. When employee stress is reduced, the staff are more likely to do their best, and, as a result, the residents receive quality, person-centered care and service.

In "What a difference management makes!", Eaton mapped out the vicious cycle of turnover and identified understaffed shifts as a root cause. As she described the problem, turnover leads to understaffed shifts, which cause stress. Staff working under stressful conditions make errors: they skip steps in important processes of care, their judgment is eroded, and they are more likely to get hurt trying to do things by themselves because co-workers do not have time to help. To make matters worse, under the stress of delivering rushed, harried care, staff relations deteriorate. CNAs snap at one another, and nurses issue orders without consideration of tone. As a result, call-outs[1] and turnover increase, perpetuating the vicious cycle (see Figure 3.1).

When a home is consistently understaffed, clinical outcomes suffer. As CNAs have reported to researchers—and we have learned through personal experience—range-of-motion exercises are often skipped and assistance with drinking and eating can be rushed when staff are working short-staffed. In many facilities, CNAs often skip residents' showers when they're stretched too thin trying to care for too many residents.

Let's look at the ramifications of skipping a resident's shower due to working understaffed. In most facilities, CNAs complete a thorough assessment of residents' skin during their shower to check for changes and the early detection of decubitus ulcers or other skin issues. In many traditional nursing homes, residents receive two showers a week according to a set schedule. If a facility is understaffed for two of a resident's shower days in a row, she may go 10 days without a full body check, and a skin issue could develop unnoticed. Staffing issues in nursing homes always affect care outcomes for residents.

Quality of life is likewise affected when staff are stressed and must rush care. During the Quality Partners of Rhode Island Center for Medicare/Medicaid Services–funded national pilot with 254 nursing

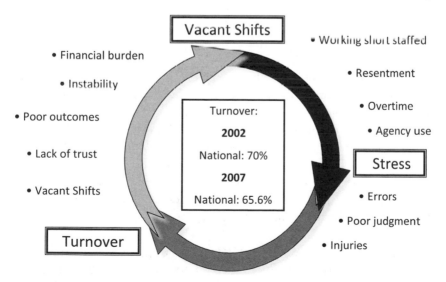

Figure 3.1.
Eaton's Vicious Cycle of Vacant Shifts, Stress, and Turnover. Copyright © 2010 B&F Consulting, Inc., and David J. Farrell.

homes focused on workforce retention, corporate executives were asked to interview their CNAs about what it was like to work understaffed. One CNA said, "Hectic! Fingernails don't get clipped, men don't get shaved, and people are left with empty cups." Another simply said, "Hell."

The executives also asked what it was like to work fully staffed. One CNA said, "You can do the little things for the residents, like give them a hug." Another said: "You can give them a back rub, talk with them. I can take the time to be more human." In other words, when this CNA works understaffed, she has to shut down some of her humanity, and the compassion that comes with it, because she has to rush to try to meet so many people's minimum needs during her shift.

Burnout is a major issue for many CNAs, who, when they consistently work understaffed, can become overwhelmed by the cries of residents, the complaints of families, and the need to "hurry up." They learn to shut down their emotions and close their heart in order to get through the basic tasks of the day. Yet this goes against their "intrinsic motivation to care" as Eaton puts it. CNAs come to this work with open hearts and don't want to stay in a job that doesn't allow them to work caringly. Organizations thrive when they support their CNAs and help them avoid burnout, and that starts with how they schedule their staff and respond to absenteeism. Eaton found that it is what leaders do that has the biggest impact on staff attendance.

The Elements of an Effective Approach

Believe it or not, employee absenteeism is not a universal or insoluble problem. There are a number of evidence-based best practices that leaders can implement to reduce call-outs and achieve stable attendance. It is a complex organizational problem, though, and requires a multifaceted plan of action to reduce absenteeism and understaffed shifts. Just as Eaton's vicious cycle notes that absences and turnover generate more absences and more turnover, so too, when homes support attendance, their initial stability creates more stability. One of the best ways to improve teamwork within an organization is to improve attendance.

It starts with a good quality improvement process: collect data on attendance and then conduct a careful root cause analysis of all the possible issues before deciding on the interventions that would work best to address the specific causes in your facility.[2]

Some attendance problems are the direct result of a leader's failure to consistently do the things that reduce employee absenteeism. The key word there is *consistently*. Most administrators tackle absenteeism when it becomes an unavoidable burden and address the issues by punishing the staff calling out the most. They address the issue on the individual employee level but do not address the organizational root causes.

The basic elements of a comprehensive approach to sustained good attendance are as follows:

- Collect accurate and comprehensive attendance data.

- Adopt and implement clear, fair, and flexible attendance policies and practices that provide both a sympathetic understanding of staff's problems and accountability for meeting commitments.

- Reward reliability and good attendance instead of paying bonuses for taking last-minute assignments.

- Make it a priority to prevent understaffed shifts and use an All-Hands-on-Deck approach to help out if a shift is understaffed so that you do not exhaust those staff and generate call-outs for the next day.

- Develop a stable staffing schedule so people know what they can count on. Post the staffing schedule in a clear, easy-to-read format, well in advance of the beginning of each month, and provide a copy of the schedule to every employee on the schedule.

- Develop clear systems and forms for staff to switch shifts and make other schedule changes.

- Maintain steady daily staffing hours.

- Use regular eight-hour shifts rather than long "Baylor" shifts.

- Use consistent assignments.

Collect Accurate Attendance Data Daily and Share It with Staff

Leaders tend to assess attendance based on their subjective impressions. Ask an administrator about absenteeism, and chances are you'll hear something like, "Not bad, we only had two call-outs last weekend. That's an improvement for us." In a profession so geared to monitoring clinical trends (e.g., pressure ulcer rate, restraint rate) to determine whether a system is breaking down, it is surprising how little attention is given to attendance data, although attendance can have a profound impact on clinical trends, and the data are relatively easy to collect.

Tracking and reporting attendance shows that management is serious about it and helps you retain high-performing, reliable nurses and CNAs. Everyone knows that we count what matters. Homes have been able to have better attendance just by including in the paychecks an accounting of each staff member's attendance. When attendance is monitored, employees with good attendance feel reassured to know that leadership is doing something to prevent understaffed shifts. High performers will not tolerate the low performance of their peers. As another job becomes available, they will leave a home plagued by call-outs and understaffing. High performers want to work with other high performers in a stable work environment.

People need to be reminded consistently that their commitment to arrive to work on time as scheduled is deeply valued by the organization. One effective way to demonstrate that is to publicly reward employees with excellent attendance records. Attendance should be discussed at every general staff meeting. In his community meetings, Farrell presented data such as total number of call-outs, the number of staff with perfect attendance, and the percentage of shifts worked fully staffed. Every month, he reminded staff why stability is critical to resident care and service. He shared attendance data whenever quality care measures were discussed, reinforcing the causal relationship between stable staffing and quality care. He emphasized the connection between stability and a quality work environment.

In tracking attendance data, it is important to collect data for every employee in each department. Usually, having one person (and one backup) coding and tracking attendance works best. All call-out slips should go to this individual, who documents call-outs on each employee's attendance record. This individual should track individual and facility trends by day of the week, by unit, and by shift, as well as documenting the total number of call-outs per month. By collecting and monitoring these attendance data for the organization, as opposed to only measuring each individual's attendance, the leaders are more likely to determine whether their interventions are effective.

It is critically important for the person who collects attendance data to input call-outs as they occur, reviewing attendance records in the process. That way, they can alert supervisors to trends, making a copy of employees' attendance records and sending them to their supervisors as issues are identified. Providing timely feedback to the employee is key. If an employee has a rash of absences, check in with the person immediately to understand what is happening and see what you can do to help.

Another best practice is to give employees regular and consistent feedback regarding their own attendance by making a copy of each employee's attendance record on a quarterly basis and including it in his or her paycheck. Use three basic form letters that can be modified as needed to accompany the employee's attendance record. The first letter is for employees with good attendance. It thanks them for being reliable and for honoring their commitment to the residents and the facility. Include a small gift card in this letter. The second letter is for employees with satisfactory attendance. It indicates that their attendance is acceptable but leaves room for improvement. The third letter is for employees with an attendance problem. It lets them to know that their supervisor will be talking with them about their attendance. As with any feedback, these letters and attendance records work best when they are delivered consistently and promptly. When employees know that you are counting their attendance, they are more mindful about it. It is human nature.

Help Staff Overcome Barriers to Attendance

Leaders should decide in advance how many absences will trigger an intervention and alert staff when they are approaching that number, rather than wait for a violation of the attendance policy. The resulting intervention should be offered not for disciplinary reasons but to express concern for the welfare of the employee.

The first meeting should take the form of a conversation to explore the factors affecting attendance and whether any adjustments or assistance from the organization can help the staff member solve the problem(s) causing the lapses in their attendance. Expressing genuine care and concern for the employee's well-being goes a long way toward gaining trust. Here are some questions to consider asking:

- Would a different schedule help?

- Is the shift not working?

- Are there some days where it is harder to get here than others?

- Would you be better able to come in if you were working fewer shifts?
- Are there other issues that are contributing to absences?
- How are relations with your supervisor and co-workers?
- How can we be of assistance?

Leaders must also seek out staff who have improved their attendance and let them know that their efforts are appreciated. This serves as strong reinforcement for the employees, who may have had to make significant efforts to be reliable and dependable in their attendance. Acknowledging these efforts soon after seeing an improvement helps prevent employees from slipping back.

In Eaton's study, a pervasive sentiment among the leaders of high-absenteeism and high-turnover facilities was—"their personal life is not my problem." Leaders in low-turnover homes had the opposite attitude, and it showed in the way they treated the employees with poor attendance.

Low-wage employees struggle to make ends meet without much cushion to handle extra expenses related to illness, child care, transportation, or even basic shelter. Such everyday struggles can present challenges that affect attendance and likely have an adverse impact in their ability to manage day-to-day responsibilities outside of work. Facing these challenges can take a toll on a person's self-esteem. Leaders understand that when obstacles keep an employee from work, the employee is a person with problems, not a problem person. When employers help employees who are good at their job solve off-the-job barriers to attendance, by offering assistance such as short-term loans or other interventions, staff develop a deep commitment and loyalty to their employer.

Connie McDonald, the administrator at Maine General Rehabilitation and Nursing Care in Augusta, Maine, put it like this: "Many who work in long-term care have hard lives. I want this job to be a place of stability for them. I hope it can anchor life for them."

Another administrator told us: "We're dealing with their problems because they're dealing with their problems. It is just a question of whether we deal with them up front or we force staff underground with what they are dealing with. When we force their issues underground, we wind up dealing with the problems in other ways, when they can't come to work, or are carrying their worries without any help or recognition from us as their employer. That's when we can lose a good worker who's having a bad time of it."

Employee assistance programs (EAPs) offer assistance with enrolling in income supports, mental health counseling, legal support and referrals, and an array of other services that many low-wage earners typically do not have access to. An EAP usually covers not only staff members, but also everyone in their household. So, if a CNA has a son with a drug dependence issue, the CNA can access help through the EAP. An EAP is a cost-effective investment because the annual cost is typically less than the estimated $2,500 it can cost to replace a CNA. An effectively utilized EAP can help employees overcome the difficulties that keep them from getting to the job—or, ultimately, staying in it.

The No-Fault Attendance Policy

Some facilities have adopted a no-fault attendance policy that takes the guesswork out of trying to judge the legitimacy of an absence. Under this policy, all absences are treated the same. There is no classification of absences as either "excused" or "not excused." Absences are simply counted, not qualified.

At first glance, it may appear that a no-fault policy conveys that leaders don't care why their employees call out. But in fact, it is a solid approach to building goodwill and trust by acknowledging that your employees are adults with lives outside of work. This approach promotes fairness and trust and takes the managers out of the uncomfortable position of having to assess the legitimacy of an absence.

When employees won't be judged for their reason for calling out, they are more likely to tell managers the real reason why they can't get to work. And when managers learn about the challenges their employees face, they can counsel their employees in how to overcome those challenges or refer them to the EAP.

The key is for managers to approach attendance from a quality improvement perspective, asking, "how can we make this better?" The no-fault attendance policy takes away the punitive nature of judging attendance. Is the employee otherwise a valued contributor to your organization? For staff who can be counted on when they are here, figure out how to count on them to be here. You can only do that together. If staff are not dependable contributors on the job, then there are other reasons to terminate their employment.

The no-fault attendance policy calls for simply keeping track of call-outs and addressing employees when they exceed a standard number (e.g., three in a 90-day period). Any time an employee is absent unexpectedly is cause for notice. Several instances in a relative short period of time, or repeated unpredictable absences over a longer period are worthy of inquiry. In a meeting with someone whose absences you're concerned about, a no-fault policy allows you to find out why, whether it is something that can be expected to continue, if there is any help that can be offered, and how to have them in the schedule realistically, so co-workers are not caught short by their inability to be there. No-fault policies will only work if they are accompanied by fact-based decision making and caring interventions. When the number of absences reaches the limit or a red flag, honest discussion and constructive interventions should be the first step, not discipline.

It is important to handle requests for time off from staff effectively. Farrell recounts in his journal finding a glitch in the process for approving requests for time off and then scheduling the time off. The scheduler didn't receive notice of the approval and put people on the schedule on days they were approved to be off. The result was a perception by the staff that management did not care. He had to revise the process to make sure that everyone was in the loop. Fixing the glitch helped both to stabilize the schedule and to minimize systems errors that made staff perceive the management as uncaring.

Any scheduling system must be able to accommodate reasonable requests for time off. Allowances should be made for one-time or rare events. Staffing coordinators should understand their responsibility to work supportively with an employee who is requesting a day off rather than responding by simply restating scheduling policies. If staff have the need for the day off and it is denied them, they will still have the need and will likely take the day off as an unplanned absence. As a result, even though they had informed the staffing coordinator of their need for a day off, their absense is not planned for or scheduled for, and instead the nursing supervisor has to deal with it at the last minute. This increases the likelihood that the assignment will go unfilled, leading to an understaffed shift.

An effective scheduling process also allows for employees to arrange to cover for each other. Having a system where people can trade days off is good because it allows staff to help each other out. Utilize the usual rules governing worker-initiated changes in schedules, including limits on overtime, written documentation of the agreement, and holding the originally scheduled employee responsible for the substitute's attendance. If someone consistently needs time off at the last minute, a timely discussion to help the person manage life circumstances or to shift from full-time to per diem status may be in order.

Use Bonuses to Reward Good Attendance

Perfect attendance bonuses have also been shown to motivate staff to improve attendance. Some administrators hold a reliability raffle every few months for all employees who have had excellent attendance. The prize may be a day off with pay—a gift that reliable people value highly. Another option is bonuses for people whose attendance is perfect or excellent within a certain time period. The time period must be relatively short—a month or a pay period works well—because it becomes too difficult for people not to miss a single day over too long a time, and you want the bonus to be attainable enough to act as an effective incentive. This is important. If a bonus is unattainable, it is an ineffective incentive. If no one is getting your bonuses, then you should consider changing your incentives. A popular bonus is a lump sum payment (e.g., $25 for a month), or a boost in the employee's hourly rate for the next pay period (e.g., $0.25 more per hour). A gift such as a gas card or grocery card is also a good incentive. This may seem costly, but it is an invaluable investment in your reliable staff, and far less costly than the overtime or bonus pay driven by absenteeism. It will reduce the stress that absences create and provide a boost as you express positive appreciation for a character trait you value—dependability.

On the other hand, the practice of paying a significant hourly bonus to staff for taking a last-minute assignment when there is an unscheduled or unexpected absence creates many problems. For instance, staff who reliably come to work as scheduled receive less pay than those who take last-minute assignments. Also,

- Scheduled staff never know who they'll be working with.

- The stress and the financial inequity can cause full-time staff to opt to switch to per diem, so they can wait for those last-minute assignment bonus calls.

- Staff can become more casual about their attendance, figuring that if they miss a shift, they can always pick up another shift later in the week and potentially earn more money that week by doing so.

Rather than amplifying the chaos and instability caused by frequent call-outs by paying a bonus to last-minute replacements, give the extra pay to the reliable people who work a regular schedule and provide great care and service each day. Scott West did this (see Chapter 5), and by making full-time and guaranteed part-time hours a better financial deal than filling in at the last minute, he reduced call-outs.

Another proven method for improving attendance is combining attendance and longevity incentives. Under this system, anyone who earns an attendance bonus in any time period is eligible for a cumulative bonus at the end of the year. For example, for each month someone earns a perfect attendance bonus, they can be given a bonus amount that is banked for them and can be collected in December. Or someone with perfect attendance for an entire quarter can get an extra paid day off. Paying cash for some or all of an employee's unused sick time at the end of the calendar year is another effective incentive.

In addition to individual rewards, rewarding a group of co-workers on a shift, department, or unit/neighborhood that has the fewest shifts worked short in a given month or pay period helps everyone pull together.

Incentives will only work if there are clear rules for eligibility. Staff need to work every shift they are scheduled for, and to be on time. However, staff should not be disqualified for absences that cause supervisors to hesitate. Their hesitation usually means they feel the reason for the absence was one that was not within the control of the employee and that an exception should be made. Again, discretion is called for here, and fairness is essential. If people know you would make that exception for anyone, they will trust the process.

Fairness is crucial in scheduling and in awarding attendance bonuses. If staff experiences favoritism in scheduling practices—if some are not accommodated when they need days off, for instance, while others are—they'll resent attendance bonuses as unfair, and a good incentive program will be undermined.

Be Transparent and Flexible in Your Scheduling Practices

Staff scheduling practices can either help or hinder absenteeism. Susan Eaton found that work schedules were a critical factor in the lives of CNAs and nurses, both on and off the job. Work schedules dictate how other aspects of life are handled: doctor appointments, meetings with teachers, and so forth. Here too, she identified significant differences between the scheduling practices in *low-* versus *high-turnover* facilities.

Eaton classified homes according to whether their schedules were rigid or flexible. The facilities that used flexibility in their scheduling had the least absenteeism and the lowest turnover. She found that these leaders considered the personal lives of the frontline staff when dealing with call-offs, showing compassion and concern for employee well-being when staff called out and reaching out later to help the employee solve the problem if necessary.

In the rigidly scheduled, *high-turnover* homes, managers made it clear through word and action that they had little concern for the staff and their welfare, and absenteeism rates were high. This became a vicious cycle, as leaders faced with rising call-outs became even more rigid, tightening the rules and instituting disciplinary actions.

Eaton found that schedules in *low-turnover* facilities were posted well in advance, giving staff members sufficient notice of their schedule and any open shifts or changes to the schedule. Knowing which residents they were caring for and which staff they were working with let employees know who was counting on them. This is a good organizational practice. The more that the employer can provide systemic stability, the more the workplace and workforce respond in kind. Stability then breeds stability.

In Eaton's study, the staff in the *high-turnover* homes viewed the scheduling procedures as haphazard and chaotic. Changes were made to the schedule without sufficient notice—and often, from the staff's point of view, without justification. Staff scheduling was clearly not a priority for the leaders, and was often delegated to a receptionist or a CNA on light duty following an injury. Scheduling employees is time consuming and takes organizational skills. Putting someone in this position with little or no training is a clear demonstration of the low value scheduling has for management, while the reality is that it has a serious negative impact on the affected staff. Farrell regards the staff scheduler as one of the key positions in the home.

The lesson here is to have a clear scheduling process that everyone can rely on and understands. Staff members need to be informed of their schedule in a timely manner. The master monthly schedule should be posted well in advance of the start of a new month (preferably 10 days ahead), with clear guidelines regarding how to sign up for any available shifts. It should be easy to read. Copies should be provided for each employee on the schedule. If the schedule needs to be changed for any reason, individuals need to be informed well ahead of time. Finally, all forms for schedule changes and time off should be easy to use and readily available.

If the process is consistent, people will come to trust the reliability of the scheduling process. They can make their plans and take care of their lives outside of work. They know when they are being counted on. Having stable staffing starts with having a stable schedule.

Choose Your Staffing Coordinators Wisely and Support Them Well

The role of staffing coordinator merits special consideration.

Many staffing coordinators are harassed 24/7 and get little thanks for their efforts to get a full complement of staff on every shift, every unit, every day. They are constantly bombarded as they patch the schedule together and fill shifts, only to start all over when they receive the next call-out.

It is interesting to note that both the *high-* and *low-turnover* facilities in Eaton's study had full-time staffing coordinators, but Eaton found vast differences in the staffing practices between the two sets of homes in her study. Eaton observed that staffing coordinators wield a tremendous amount of power, so they should be carefully selected. They need excellent organizational skills, math skills, and interpersonal skills. If the staffing coordinator appears to play favorites, always setting up certain people for overtime shifts or giving them first choice in days off, the morale of the facility will sink.

Staffing coordinators need support and one-on-one education from facility administrators in order to successfully prevent understaffing. Farrell regularly met with his staffing coordinator and arranged for regular meetings with nursing leadership, thereby ensuring that she felt like an important part of the team. Every Tuesday, right after the stand-up meeting, she joined Farrell and his nursing leadership team to discuss the staff and staffing, bringing both the current and future month's schedules. Farrell and the team reviewed the schedules and looked at overtime data together. They talked about how to cover for somebody's vacation time, how new staff were settling in, what if any changes were needed to people's consistent assignment, and hiring needs. As time went on and effective and flexible staffing practices were put into place and sustained, these meetings became a positive experience for everyone around the table. "We got energized by the positive HR data we were looking at, and it motivated us to keep up what we were doing and it encouraged us to always be looking for ways that we could do more," Farrell says.

Don't De-motivate Your Employees

In *Hardwiring Excellence*, Quint Studer reminds us, "The problem is not motivation. It is the ways we unintentionally de-motivate employees." The quality of the work environment is a a big factor in attendance. When supervisors do not "see" their people, staff feel as though they are invisible to these supervisors, and that feeling is a root cause of attendance problems. Feeling invisible leaves employees feeling under-valued, and it damages their self-esteem, which can sometimes be quite damaged already by life's hardships. Mary Lescoe-Long and Michael Long (1998) described the "lack of a causal link between effort and success" that is imprinted when people have experienced prolonged severe socioeconomic disadvantage. When this is reinforced by inter-personal dynamics in the workplace, it can add stress and increase the disconnect for staff.

People want to feel like they matter. Long-term-care employees want to feel important and needed. It is hard to show up on time every day when no one seems to care whether you show up at all. One of the most effective ways to motivate a nursing home employee to come to work as scheduled is to let the person know they were missed the day they return after calling out. When an employee returns to work after a call-out and no one says anything, it can seem as if no one really cares whether they come to work or not. However, if supervisors and co-workers acknowledge their absence, it shows they matter.

With a no-fault attendance policy in place, employees are more likely to tell their supervisor the "real" reason why they called out. With that reason in hand, supervisors can immediately speak with their employees after a call-out in a spirit of *care and concern*. They will be able to say something like, "We missed you yesterday and, of course, the residents did too. I understand your son was ill. Is he all right now?"

If supervisors know their staff and the challenges they face, they can anticipate when a staff member may need a break. For example, a supervisor who hears that something happened to an employee or the employee's family can call and offer time off. This gesture goes a long way toward building loyalty and trust. In addition, the staff member, being so grateful for the gesture, may return to work sooner than expected.

Some reasons for calling out are likely to lead to several days off the schedule, not just one. In such cases, calling staff at home to find out if they may need additional days off can prevent understaffed shifts the next day (and the day after that). In the spirit of care and concern for the employees, supervisors should call employees who called off at home, ask how they are doing, and find out if they think they will be back for their next scheduled shift. The caller should make it clear that they are not calling to spy on the employee but to check on their welfare and try to prevent an understaffed shift. This allows the nursing home to proactively anticipate vacant shifts and fill them before the call-off occurs.

Loren Salvietti's Attendance Policy

The policy Loren Salvietti instituted in 2008 is presented in Box 3.1. Since it went into effect, she has dramatically reduced terminations. The example in Box 3.2 was developed by the authors to give the reader a sample policy.

Box 3.1
Attendance, Tardiness, and No-Call/ No-Show Policy
Quaboag on the Common, West Brookfield, MA, 2008

Policy: Quaboag on the Common will ensure that this facility is staffed at a level consistent with the provision of an exceptionally high level of services to our residents. For the purposes of interpreting the following procedure, an incident of absence is defined as any time an employee fails to report to work for scheduled work day(s). *Note:* The facility will pay for five sick days a year.

If an employee is going to be absent from work the employee must notify her/his supervisor or the staff scheduler by telephone each day that the employee is absent, unless other arrangements have been previously approved. Messages left on voice mail are not allowed. If an employee knows in advance that he or she will be absent, is able to arrange for a replacement, and notifies the supervisor and/or staff scheduler in writing of this arrangement, the employee will not be considered absent. In the event that the designated replacement does not work, the replacement employee calling out will be considered to be absent.

Box 3.1 *continued*

Personal Days: Each employee has the option of using two personal days per year. These two days are treated as excused absences. Under this policy employees are not required to inform their supervisor of the reason for their request for a personal day. Requests for a personal day must be submitted in writing at least 24 hours before the personal day or it will be treated as an absence. Personal days may not be taken the day before, the day of, or the day after a holiday. If you take a personal day during a weekend, you must make up that day the next weekend or as needed by the facility. Personal days are unpaid, unless the employee wishes to use vacation time to receive payment. Request for use of vacation time to receive payment for a personal day must be made in writing.

Perfect Attendance: Perfect attendance is defined as coming to work each and every day for which an employee is scheduled. (Bereavement days are excluded. Please see facility bereavement attendance policy.) If an employee knows in advance that he or she will be absent, is able to arrange for a replacement, and notifies in writing the supervisor and/or staff scheduler of this arrangement, the employee will not be considered absent and will still be considered for perfect attendance. All hourly employees with perfect attendance for four months will receive a bonus check at the end of the fourth month equal to one day's pay. All hourly employees with perfect attendance for a year will receive an additional 1% added to their annual raise.

Mandatory Leave of Absence: Any employee who is absent for more than five consecutively scheduled workdays must request a leave of absence. The request for a leave of absence must be in writing and must include the reason for the request, the start date, and an anticipated date when the employee will return to work.

The Small Necessities Leave Act: The Small Necessities Leave Act mandates that this facility provides up to 24 hours of unpaid leave during any 12-month period to "eligible employees." This leave is in addition to the 12 weeks already allowed under the Federal Family and Medical Leave Act. The employee must have been employed for at least 12 months by the employer from whom the leave is requested, and must have provided at least 1,250 hours of service for the employer during the immediately previous 12-month period. The 24-hour unpaid

Box 3.1 *continued*

leave may be taken for any of the following reasons: to participate in a parent–teacher conference or interview for a new school, to accompany a son or daughter to a doctor's appointment, or to accompany an elderly relative to a health-related appointment. Requests should be made in writing.

Excessive Absences: Any employee who has more than three incidents of absences in a 90-day period will be considered to have excessive absences. A meeting with your supervisor will take place to review your attendance. In an effort to provide consistent, reliable care to our residents and a reasonable workload to our team members, your scheduled hours over the next 90 days will be adjusted. For example, if you have been scheduled to work 37.5 hours a week and have called out excessively, your scheduled hours will be changed to 30 hours. If your attendance improves at the end of the 90-day period, you may request an increase in your scheduled hours or you may continue to work 30 hours.

Raises are given to recognize experience, good work, and loyalty to the facility. Five or more absences in a rolling calendar year will be considered when calculating your raise. One percent of your raise is based on your attendance history for the year.

Notification: Call-outs *cannot* be left on voice mail. All employees *must* speak directly to the staff scheduler, the appropriate shift coordinator, or their supervisor. An employee who leaves a call-out on voice mail will be subject to a written final warning.

Employees must notify their supervisor that they will be absent *at least 2 hours* before the start of the scheduled shift. *Please note*: For the day shift (7:00 a.m.–3:00 p.m.), *a one-hour* notice is required.

Failure to notify the supervisor in accordance with this policy will result in the employee being ineligible for sick pay for that day or days.

Weekend/Holiday Call-Outs: Employees who call out on a weekend will be required to work the following weekend or at the discretion of the department head. Employees who call out on a weekend are prohibited from replacing themselves with another employee on their makeup weekend. They are required to work the makeup weekend themselves. Employees who call out on a holiday for which they are assigned to work will be required to work on the next holiday. Employees

Box 3.1 *continued*

who call out on a holiday are prohibited from replacing themselves with another employee on their makeup holiday. They are required to work the makeup holiday themselves. Employees must work their scheduled days before and after a holiday in order to receive their holiday pay.

Tardiness: Every employee must report to work on time each scheduled workday. Employees are expected to report to their designated work areas immediately after punching in for work. Employees shall remain at their designated work area until the end of their scheduled shift except for authorized break times. Upon completion of their shift, they may leave their work area to go to the time clock to punch out. For the purpose of this policy, being marked tardy three times or quitting early three times equal an absence. If you arrange for your own coverage (i.e., call a friend to report to work early so that you may leave early), you will not be considered to have left work early.

No Call/No Show: Any employees who fail to report to work for a scheduled shift who have not notified their supervisor in accordance with the notification section of this policy (no call/no show) will be disciplined. The first no call/no show will result in a final written warning. A second no call/no show will result in termination. The termination will be effective immediately and will be processed as a voluntary resignation on the basis of job abandonment.

Erasing Absences: The opportunity to erase absences by picking up extra shifts will be offered to the staff at the discretion of the administrator based on staffing needs. Staff who pick up an extra shift and have no absences to erase may bank the erase to be used at a future date.

Box 3.2
Sample Attendance Policy

Subject: Attendance, Tardiness, and No-Call/No-Show Policy
Policy Statement: _____ **Care Center** will comply
with all state and federal regulations as they pertain to staffing levels.

Absence: An absence is defined as any time an employee fails to
report to work as scheduled, regardless of the reason given. There is no
distinction between excused or unexcused absences. All absences for
any reason are treated equally.

Notification: Any employees who are going to be absent must notify
their supervisor, the staff scheduler, or the appropriate shift coordinator
by phone *each day* that they are absent, unless other arrangements have
been previously approved. Messages left on voice mail are not allowed.

Call-outs *cannot* be left on voice mail. All employees *must* speak
directly to the staff scheduler, the appropriate shift coordinator, or their
supervisor. An employee who leaves a call-out on voice mail will be
subject to disciplinary action up to and including termination.

Employees must notify their supervisor that they will be absent *at
least 2 hours* before the start of the scheduled shift.

Weekend/Holiday Call-Outs: Employees who call out on a weekend
will be required to work the following weekend or another weekend at
the discretion of the department head. Employees who call out on a
weekend are prohibited from replacing themselves with another employee on their makeup weekend. They are required to work the makeup
weekend themselves. Employees who call out on a holiday, for which
they are assigned to work, will be required to work on the next holiday. Employees who call out on a holiday are prohibited from replacing
themselves with another employee on their makeup holiday. They are
required to work the makeup holiday themselves. Employees must work
their scheduled days before and after a holiday unless an absence on
either day is approved in advance by their supervisor in order to receive
their holiday pay.

Excessive Absences: Any employee who has more than three absences in a 90-day period (unless there are extenuating circumstances)
will be considered to have excessive absences. A meeting with your supervisor will take place to review your attendance. In an effort to provide consistent, reliable care to our residents and a reasonable workload
to our team members your scheduled hours over the next 90 days may
be adjusted at the discretion of your supervisor. For example, if you have
been scheduled to work 37.5 hours a week and have called out exces-

Box 3.2 *continued*

sively, your scheduled hours may be changed to 30 hours. If your attendance improves at the end of the 90-day period, you may request an increase in your scheduled hours or you may continue to work 30 hours. Continued excessive absenteeism will result in disciplinary action up to and including termination.

No Call/No Show: Any employees who fail to report to work for a scheduled shift who have not notified their supervisor in accordance with the notification section of this policy (no call/no show) will be disciplined. The first no call/no show will result in a final written warning. A second no call/no show will result in termination. If you fail to report for work without notification to your supervisor for three consecutive days, the company will consider that you have abandoned your employment and have voluntarily terminated the employment relationship. The termination will be effective immediately and will be processed as a voluntary resignation on the basis of job abandonment.

Tardiness: Employees are expected to be ready to start and end work on schedule. Accordingly, arriving late or leaving early in connection with scheduled work times, breaks, or meal periods is impermissible. Repeated incidents of tardiness or leaving work early may result in disciplinary action up to and including termination.

Perfect attendance: Perfect attendance is defined as coming to work each and every scheduled day (bereavement days are excluded—please see facility bereavement policy). Employees who know in advance that they will be absent are able to arrange for a replacement, and if the supervisor, staff scheduler, and/or appropriate shift coordinator is notified in writing of this arrangement, the employees will still be considered to have perfect attendance for purposes of the perfect attendance rewards. All hourly employees with perfect attendance for each month will be included in the perfect attendance raffle. Each month, winners will receive a day off with pay as the reward.

All hourly employees with perfect attendance for the year prior to their annual review may receive an additional 1% added to their annual raise in recognition of their efforts to contribute to the superior care of our residents and the success of the facility. Poor attendance will negatively impact your raise.

Name   Date

Signature

Notes

1. In different regions of the country, nursing homes use variations on this term, including call-offs, call-ins, and call-outs. We use *call-out* to mean someone who calls shortly before the shift to say they cannot come to work—an unplanned absence.

2. The Fishbone Diagram is an excellent way to visualize the root causes. This quality improvement tool has been used for years to drill down into clinical problems.

## CHAPTER 4

A Positive Chain of Leadership

Supervision

AT THE HEART OF DAVID FARRELL's success as an administrator was his trust and respect for his employees. They felt it and responded in kind, treating each other and the residents with more respect and consideration. When staff work well together, care improves, the day goes better for the residents as well as the staff, and the nursing home thrives. It all starts with good supervision, which creates what Susan Eaton called "a positive chain of leadership throughout the organization."

This chapter identifies essential elements of good supervision that are easy to put into practice and have been proven to be the foundation for good organizational performance.

Ready or Not, You're a Supervisor

In long-term care as in many other fields, the Peter Principle is alive and well when it comes to filling management positions. People get promoted to a position with a supervisory component not necessarily because they are good supervisors, but because they are good in their chosen area of expertise, which has nothing to do with supervision. Nurses who are very good at nursing wind up supervising certified nursing assistants (CNAs), even though they may have received little or no training in how to be a supervisor and may not even have an interest in supervising other people. No wonder so many of them struggle with their supervisory responsibilities.

In their 1998 study on how to improve staff retention in Kansas nursing homes, researchers Dr. Michael Long and Dr. Mary Lescoe-Long, two psychologists, found that managers and supervisors lacked critical supervisory skills even in homes that were highly regarded in their professional associations and in their communities. This is a serious problem because, as the Kansas researchers and others have found, poor supervision is one of the key causes of the high turnover and absenteeism among nurses and CNAs. High turnover and absenteeism are leading causes of poor care. Conversely, good supervisory skills can be one of the most important factors in stabilizing staffing and enabling staff to work well together for good outcomes.

On the most basic level, it is hard to establish the caring relationships that are so important to good teamwork and residents' well-being if homes continually experience newly hired CNAs and nurses leaving after just a few weeks or months. High turnover and frequent unscheduled absences are a strain on the nursing staff who remain. They must constantly train and support new co-workers. They may often find themselves "working short," caring for extra residents until a vacant position is filled. It is very hard, when working short, to provide the individual attention that makes their job meaningful and boosts the quality of residents' lives. (See Chapters 2 and 3 for more information on retaining newly hired staff and reversing absenteeism.)

When people with poor supervisory skills are made responsible for the actions of others, they often react in one of two ways. If they don't have much confidence in, or respect for, the people who report to them, or feel uncomfortable in their own role as supervisor, they are likely to rule with a heavy hand. They tend to insist that everyone follow the rules rather than taking the time to look at the reasoning behind the rules, or trying to find out what is preventing an employee from performing at his or her best. New supervisors are quite often at this end of the spectrum, because they may feel overwhelmed or intimidated by the role.

At the other end of the spectrum, they may fail to hold people to a high standard, bending over backward to accommodate staff—and then feeling taken advantage of and getting soured on the individual or on their own role as a supervisor. They may even abdicate their supervisory responsibilities altogether to focus on their other duties, tuning out the escalating chaos around them.

Whether a supervisor ignores a problem or tries to correct it in a way that comes across as tyrannical, the inappropriate action is likely to continue. This creates a vicious cycle that generates further negativity and leaves good employees without the support they need. When staff who are working hard and responsibly see that the supervisor is ineffective, they tend to "hunker down" and focus narrowly on their own area of responsibility, giving up on the possibility of a good working environment.

Good supervision has little to do with being a strict disciplinarian or finding a kind way to give negative feedback. Good supervision actually starts with trusting people and being open and available to them. It is about creating conditions that allow staff to perform at their best and expecting the best of them. It is about building and maintaining good relationships with the people you supervise. Doing so sets off a positive cycle as people develop good working relationships with each other and come together as a team to face the challenges of the day.

Bring Out the Best in Each Employee

Good supervisors are people developers. They tune in to the people they supervise. Just as good resident care starts with an individual assessment of strengths and needs, good supervision depends on getting to know who an employee is, what strengths that employee brings to the work, and where he or she might need additional guidance and benefit from developmental support. Working from that basis of knowledge and focusing on positive growth, a good supervisor can customize his or her approach to supervision to bring out the best in each employee.

Supervisors who expect the best from people and help them achieve it wind up with higher productivity and happier staff. This goodwill builds on itself, like a bank account with compound interest: the more productive people are, the more productive and happier they become. Instead of doing what they need just to get by, they stretch to meet the next challenge. When supervisors spend more time developing people, they spend less time disciplining.

One of the best ways to understand good supervision is to think of the best supervisor you've ever had. Most likely, the one who comes to mind set high standards and then helped you achieve them. Maybe this person saw something in you before you saw it in yourself, inspiring you to strive to be your best and live up to what he or she saw.

The research about this in our field matches what researchers have found about other kinds of organizations: People thrive and perform best when their supervisors trust and support them. In its review of over 106,000 employee satisfaction surveys from nearly 2,000 homes, My InnerView, the largest organization that conducts staff and family satisfaction surveys, found that what matters most to nurses and CNAs is that their supervisors care, listen, and help reduce their job stress.

Think back to David Farrell's journal entry about the lack of clean linen in the building. Clearly, the housekeeping/laundry supervisor distrusted the CNAs. Maybe he thought they were lazy, storing linen in resident rooms to save themselves the walk to the linen closets. Maybe he thought they were dishonest, planning to take the linen home and stashing it in residents' closets to make it easier to steal without being seen. In any event, he was convinced that putting out more clean linen would only encourage their laziness or thievery. In fact, when CNAs don't trust that the organization will provide enough linen for them to meet their residents' needs, most effective CNAs do stash linen to ensure that they can do their job. Stashing linen then is an indicator of a broken linen delivery system, not of dishonest CNAs. However, by approaching such a situation with blame and distrust, managers don't fix the root cause of the problem or repair CNAs' mistrust of the system. An effective supervisor would note stashed linen as a red flag and go to bat with the laundry department to ensure that staff have the supplies they need to care for residents. This would engender CNAs' trust and open the door to problem solving when similar situations arise.

A supervisor who takes a disciplinary approach and never fixes the underlying causes of problems generates a climate of distrust, disconnection, and poor communication. A supervisor who believes that people want to do a good job will look for the cause of the problem when something goes wrong. By taking that approach, and by removing the obstacles in the path of good care, a good supervisor creates an atmosphere of mutual trust and goodwill.

Walk the Talk

Supervisors live in a fishbowl. Employees are always watching how supervisors and managers act and follow what they see. When supervisors chip in, they teach teamwork and cooperation by modeling it.

When supervisors answer call lights, they demonstrate by their actions that being helpful to any resident in need is every staff person's responsibility.

By contrast, if leaders say they want teamwork but then walk by a call bell, they are not modeling teamwork; they are modeling "not my job." John Maxwell, a noted international leadership expert, said people's minds are changed more by observation than by argument.

James Kouzes and Barry Posner, researcher authors on leadership skills, found that credibility is the foundation for effective leadership. When employees perceive their leaders as credible, they wrote in *Credibility* (pp. 31, 32) they are more likely to

- be proud to tell others they're part of the organization
- feel a strong sense of team spirit
- feel attached and committed to the organization
- see their own values as consistent with those of the organization
- have a sense of ownership of the organization.

When employees perceive their leaders to have low credibility, they are more likely to

- produce only if they're watched carefully
- be motivated primarily by money
- say good things about the organization publicly but criticize privately
- consider looking for another job if the organization experiences trouble
- feel unsupported and criticized.

Credible leaders do what they say they will do. They clarify their own beliefs and values and explain their actions. They also unify staff around shared values, so that everyone feels that they're in it together, striving to meet common goals. Credible leaders intensify their employees' commitment to shared values by living those values daily.

Farrell described community meetings in which he told the staff he was committed to supporting them and explained the importance to residents of the efforts they were making to individualize care. During his tenure at the home, he consistently spelled out what he was doing and why he was doing it. He talked passionately about the importance of community, of trust, of being there for each other. Over and over again he built trust by being the first one to trust others.

When someone defaced his inspirational messages in the elevator, he could have put up a glass wall to keep his comments protected. Instead, he wrote an open letter to the individual, asking the person to stop disrespecting everyone by jeering at their shared values. Staff cheered him on, appreciating the fact that he had followed his words about community with action. This was a shout out for better behavior done in a way that appealed to the defacer's better nature rather than expecting that the negativity could never be turned around.

When the person stopped defacing the messages it was a victory for the whole staff, demonstrating the power of the trust and shared values they had established together. But that trust started with their faith in David, who demonstrated how much he believed in that trust and those shared values when he handled the naysayer the way that he did.

Why is it so hard to do what we say we will—and fully intend to? Often, we are derailed by the pressures of the day. A director of nursing (DON) lost credibility with her nurses when she wasn't able to fit in time to work with them to help dispose of expired narcotics. The nurses had to account for the narcotics on every shift, and they resented the burden, so the DON promised repeatedly to help. When she didn't get to it, the nurses began rolling their eyes at all the promises she made. By failing to do what she'd said she would do, she lost all credibility. Staff notice what you do and don't do, and they don't forget.

Another way that credibility can be undermined is when a staff member makes a suggestion to do something differently so as to make things better. Hearing the suggestion on the fly and seeing the merit of it, a supervisor might say, "Yeah, that sounds good," and later find out that there is more involved and it is far more complex than at first glance. Not getting back to the staff member who originally made the suggestion and explaining what the complexities are may contribute to lost credibility. Even when supervisors do follow through, they sometimes don't get back to the CNA with thanks for expressing concern about a resident's condition and letting the CNA know how it was taken care of. Closing every loop like this can build credibility and make room for further discussions on the matter.

Model Honesty and Authenticity

People in authority often think they must present a veneer of having all the answers. But in fact, transparency—letting others see us as human beings—works much better than false fronts, encouraging employees to be more real with us in turn. In surveys conducted over three decades, Kouzes and Posner consistently found that the characteristics people needed most in a leader were openness and honesty. Admitting when you don't have the answers and inviting others to join you in the search frees up your employees to do the same when they are faced with a situation they don't know how to handle. Being honest encourages others to do the same.

Employees will be much more forgiving of a supervisor's mistakes, and more willing to work with him or her to make things better, if the supervisor is real with them. Remember Farrell's story about how he regretted having decided to move a resident out of a room? When he admitted the error and apologized to the resident, a CNA who overheard him offered him comfort, assured him that things had worked out just fine.

We spend far too much time at work to make it a place where we have to wear a mask. And yet masks abound in nursing homes. One administrator we worked with was telling us in sarcastic frustration that he wondered how many grandmothers one CNA could have, after hearing for the fifth time that a grandmother's death was the cause of her unscheduled absence. When he was told that this was an excuse people often offered when they didn't feel safe giving the real reason, he was surprised. He hadn't considered that her dishonesty might indicate that some CNAs in his home were unable to trust their supervisors with the truth; he just assumed it meant that this CNA was not to be trusted.

When Loren Salvietti rolled out a new attendance policy for her Massachusetts nursing home at staff meetings (for details, see Chapter 3), she started by telling her employees: "You're adults. I trust you." She then explained that she had changed the policy to accomplish two goals. Goal 1 was to be sure that they were never understaffed due to unexpected absences, because of the danger to residents and staff from understaffing. Goal 2 was to make sure that staff could attend to their needs outside of work, because she knew they all had a lot of pressures and responsibilities in their daily lives. By letting her staff in on her thinking and treating them with respect, she earned their trust and their cooperation. While she had fired 50 people for poor attendance the previous year, she only needed to terminate 1 in a year under the new approach.

CNAs have lots of good reasons to believe it is not safe to tell authority figures the truth. The Long and Lescoe-Long study explained how our experiences shape our outlook on life. A significant majority of the CNAs in their study had experienced severe economic disadvantages during their formative years. Those disadvantages often put them in situations where working hard may work to their disadvantage because of the rules of the "system." Consider the single parent who works extra hours in August to get money for school supplies for her children's return to school, only to learn that her efforts and extra earnings have made her children ineligible for health coverage through Medicaid. Those disadvantages, and the need to function outside the system's rules, continue to be the case for many who work in long-term care. The CNAs in a Massachusetts focus group led by Barbara Frank and Cathie Brady about health insurance illuminated one of the ways that living on the economic margins can give people an ingrained distrust of systems and people in authority. The one benefit of their low pay, they said, is that they and their families qualify for Medicaid-funded health care coverage. That is a blessing, since they don't earn nearly enough to cover the premiums and copays required by their employer's health insurance plan. But if they took on extra hours to pay for additional expenses now and then, like the school supplies or Christmas presents they had to buy for their kids, they risked inching over the cutoff point for Medicaid benefits and being terminated from its health care plan. The only way to protect their families, they learned, was to work "off the books" and not report the extra income. The CNAs in the Lescoe-Long study, the researchers noted, "lacked a causal link" between their efforts and successful outcomes: As hard as they work, they remain poor.

At a goodbye luncheon for an administrator who had led his nursing home for a decade, one CNA after another stood up to talk about what a genuine person the administrator was. One spoke of the administrator's concern about her family after a hurricane had devastated Haiti, where she was from and where many of her relatives still lived. Another talked about his awkwardness in trying to pronounce her name, how they had laughed about his mistakes, and the fun they had in working together to correct them because he insisted on learning how to say it fluently. She said so many other bosses she'd had had just given up and avoided using her name. That administrator's staff trusted his sincerity and genuine concern for them. They knew where he stood, and that he meant what he said. His authenticity allowed them to let down their own masks and be authentic too. With that trust, they were able to tell him the truth about their needs and realities, and he was able to make adjustments in advance instead of piecing together a schedule because he could not anticipate their absences.

Make Sure Everyone Has the Whole Picture

A common error in supervision is assuming that employees know more than they do about the supervisor's expectations, the home's goals, and the thinking behind them. Employees who don't have a clear idea of what is expected of them may know enough to do part of what is needed but not to follow through completely. And they're unlikely to ask for clarification, usually because they are unaware that they don't have a full understanding. They don't know what they don't know.

Even when employees know that they don't have the whole picture, they may not feel safe saying so. It takes a trusting relationship for an employee to let a supervisor know about a gap in understanding, and to approach a supervisor when he or she is busy. When English is not the first language of an employee, this may add to an employee's hesitation about asking for clarification. Most people just do the best they can and hope it is right.

When people know why something is important, they are far more able to do what is expected of them. In one home a nurse had an eye-opening experience after becoming a mentor for new CNAs. When she learned what the CNAs were taught in their certification training, she realized how little they were told about the aging process. She had assumed that CNA training was far more extensive than it is, and finding out the truth made her realize that they were operating under a handicap, unequipped with the knowledge needed to provide the level of care she had been expecting.

That nurse was pleasantly surprised to discover how much she could help a CNA she was mentoring by filling in gaps in her knowledge. She learned that when CNAs understood the theory behind a task and realized what a difference it made to residents, they took extra time to do the individual things each resident needed. Knowing more about aging in general, and their residents specifically, gave the CNAs more empathy, and with empathy came better care.

In *The Leadership Challenge*, Kouzes and Posner tell a story about an army experiment. Participants in a special training program went through a rigorous few weeks that culminated in a long march. On the day of the march, the soldiers were divided into four groups. Blood tests for stress indicators were taken during the march and again 24 hours later.

These soldiers were all in comparable shape with comparable ability. The only difference between the groups was how honestly and how often their leaders communicated with them.

- Group 1 was told exactly how long they had to march—20 kilometers—and they were given regular progress reports along the way.

- Group 2 was told "this is the long march you heard about." Nobody knew how far they would march, nor were they informed of their progress along the way.

- Group 3 was told they would march 15 kilometers. They were given no progress reports, and when they got to 14 kilometers, they were told they really had to march 6 more.

- Group 4 was told they had to march 25 kilometers. They too had no progress reports, and at 14 kilometers they were told they would only march 20.

So how did they do? You're probably not surprised to hear that Group 1 did best. Not only did they finish first, but they scored better in their stress indicators. It is also no surprise that Group 2 came in last. They had no information to go on and no feedback along the way. They were left in the dark, and their performance reflected it.[1]

This echoes what Susan Eaton concluded after comparing staff in high-performing/low-turnover homes with staff in low-performing/high-turnover ones. "[T]hese individuals were not fundamentally different 'kinds of people' with different 'work ethics,'" she writes of the staff in the low-turnover homes. "They were, however, acting in a different organizational and human setting, being treated differently and being trusted and valued at a much higher level." In other words, the people were not that different, but the management and supervision in the organizations where they worked were very different.

Celebrate the Good News and Brainstorm About the Bad

When staff have access to key data, understand what it means, and know how their own work affects that data, shared information can be a trigger for higher productivity and better care. When data show positive changes—fewer falls, fewer urinary tract infections, less skin breakdown—share this good news with your staff. Let them know that their hard work is making a difference. Celebrate good news, and it will multiply. Again, think of this as compound interest. The more you acknowledge it, the more it grows.

If the data are not so positive, share this as well, but frame it in an "in-it-together" manner, focusing on figuring out how to deal with this dilemma together rather than trying to assign blame. The goal is to share your clinical, human resource, and satisfaction data with your staff and help them interpret it.

Farrell had his staff establish goals as a team. To reduce falls, he held short meetings with the CNAs and nurses on each unit, looking at the data, discussing what could be causing the falls, and identifying resident-by-resident solutions. Farrell helped his nurses and staff see how they were doing and explore ways of doing better. Not only was he supporting their work as a team, he was showing them how to use their own data. When people know why they are being asked to do something and they see the benefit of it, they are more likely to follow through on the action needed. When they are asked to become part of the solution by drawing on their own expert knowledge about the people they care for, they come forward.

This was effective in part because it demonstrated his faith in his staff. caregivers, like the rest of us, thrive on positive feedback and are highly responsive to being included. It also made use of the staff's combined knowledge to come up with a better solution to the problem than Farrell could have reached on his own or in consultation with his DON. When staff are comfortable enough to engage in a root-cause analysis together, effective solutions more quickly become apparent.

But the basis for the change was the information Farrell shared with his nursing staff. When they knew what was expected of them, it was easier to set targets for themselves to do better. And they did do better, reducing the number of falls.

Feedback helps fuel performance. Just as the army found in its study of the marches, regular feedback has a physiological effect that contributes to better performance. Medical science is making remarkable discoveries about the relationship between our state of mind and our mental and physical health. Recent brain function analyses have found that positive thoughts, feelings, and expectations cause the brain to create endorphins, which in turn triggers a positive feeling in the body, an energizing outlook on life, and improved self-esteem.

In other words, the more positive your attitude and expectations, the more likely your brain is to produce substances that boost your body's power. It is another of those self-perpetuating cycles, with positive feelings engendering more of the same.

Never Underestimate the Power of Positive Feedback

For many frontline workers in long-term care, a boost of self-esteem is sorely needed. When staff get that boost and feel better about themselves, their interactions with residents get better too.

Group appreciation is good, but it is not as effective as one-on-one feedback. Think back to Farrell's story about telling a restorative nursing assistant that he noticed her positive approach and attitude. She was taken aback when he thanked her for the difference she made, saying that no one had ever said that to her before. Farrell saw her contribution and impact and let her know that he saw it. Their relationship had a different level of depth because he shared his appreciation.

Individual feedback is phenomenally powerful. In fact, it is a supervisor's most powerful tool, and as such should be employed often. A good supervisor sees the individual accomplishments and says *out loud* what was observed. When people perform in a way that is desirable, personally recognizing the action will cement it.

During a gathering of New Orleans nursing home leaders from the homes affected by Katrina a year after the hurricane, as Brady and Frank were talking about the importance of providing individual encouragement and feedback to their employees, a director of nursing told the group what her own experience of recognition had meant to her. She pulled out of her purse a card she said was among the belongings she had salvaged from her damaged home. It was a card she had received from a supervisor at the end of her first week starting out as a CNA. She read the letter out loud. Her supervisor had written about how well she had worked with the residents and her co-workers, and told the woman she was sure she would be successful as a caregiver. After reading it to the group, the woman said the card had meant the world to her because at the end of her first week she'd felt overwhelmed and unsure. Hearing that she was on the right track, had potential, and had already done well gave her the encouragement she needed to persist.

Recognition can be a card, a quiet two-minute conversation, or a public announcement. Situations and personalities will dictate what works best in the way of personal recognition. Praise is feedback that lets employees know that you see how well they are doing, and you value them for it.

Farrell studied what administrators at the highest-performing nursing homes did on a consistent basis. One practice was conducting slower rounds that focused more on people. He picked up on the importance of slowing down to connect with people and ask the right questions, realizing that building relationships with his staff is "the job."

Farrell had always conducted rounds, but never like this—never with a conscientious focus on the individuals working there. He had always connected with people. But now, with a deeper knowledge base, he was much more aware of what to ask about and what it meant to the organizational performance. His rounds were a way to encourage and appreciate people every day.

Good energy can be released with simple positive acts, and they are contagious. A news story told of a morning scene at a drive-through fast-food chain. As one customer was waiting for his coffee, the car behind started honking. When the customer paid for his coffee, he gave the cashier extra money and asked her to tell the driver behind him his coffee was paid for. The impatient driver was so chagrined and touched to have his coffee paid for, even as he had behaved so impatiently, that he in turn paid for the driver behind him. This continued through the entire line of customers in that morning rush.

Teach Staff to Think for Themselves

John C. Maxwell, in Developing the Leader Within You, asserts that the greatest avenue for growth of a company is through growing the skills of its people. He also writes that "it is better to train ten people to work than to do the work of ten people, but it is harder."

Good supervisors are always developing the abilities of those around them. Perhaps one of the most important of those abilities is critical thinking. When staff don't know why something is important, they can easily overlook it. Several Connecticut nursing homes started offering their CNAs college-level courses. Once the CNAs taking the Issues in Aging course learned how residents' sight is affected by vision changes, they had a different understanding of the importance of adjusting room light for residents and were more conscientious in doing so. They also learned how to use residents' records to learn about any vision problems their residents had, so they can figure out when and how lighting should be adjusted.

Before supervisors can effectively develop the skills of their employees, they need to develop their own. Scott West, an administrator in Burlington, Vermont, set out to build the hiring skills of his supervisors and managers. He wanted them to know how to make good hiring choices. When his director of maintenance said he didn't know how to interview, Scott used a managers' meeting to discuss good interview practices. He joined the maintenance director for the first few interviews, slowly turning more of the responsibilities over to him. His managers and supervisors learned to make good hiring decisions, which were a significant factor in Birchwood's turnaround to high retention. His managers were able to rise to meet West's expectations because he gave them the help they needed to succeed. In a similar process at her home, Loren Salvietti developed her nurse managers' hiring skills, talking through what to look for and how to interview. Her ads now direct prospective employees to the nurse in charge of the unit where the vacancy is so that nurses build their own teams on their units.

When staff begin to think critically and to make good decisions, leaders are able to focus on moving the organization ahead. A DON in Maine pointed to his clean desk as a sign of how his work life had simplified once he employed shared decision making. Before he started including his employees in decision making, his desk was always piled high with things he needed to do but never got to because he was so often pulled away to intervene in daily conflicts. "Now," he said, "I have time for looking forward instead of playing catch-up."

Including staff in decision making also opens the door to solutions that may work better than what the leader could come up with alone, and it hones staff's critical thinking skills, which will pay off later as they more easily tackle whatever challenges arise.

De-escalate Conflict

The work in long-term care is hard, physically and emotionally. It is all about people, and it involves working with a lot of very different people, every day. As a result, there are complex interpersonal dynamics in play 24/7. Tempers are bound to flare, and when they do, it is easy to get caught up in the moment. Good supervisors use their good people skills to intercede and de-escalate situations.

Long and Lescoe-Long saw how nurses' reactions could throw fuel on the fire, escalating tension and conflict between nursing assistants. They found, too, that managers were often unable to deal with people who lacked good interpersonal skills, and that was a primary cause of turnover, among both the nurses and the CNAs. Lescoe-Long noted that most nurses were very good at de-escalating situations in which residents become agitated, responding with a steady calm, but they didn't use those same skills when dealing with challenging dynamics with CNAs.

Ironically most nursing homes have conflict resolution systems in place that actually escalate conflicts. Look at how a typical nursing home handles a harsh exchange between a CNA and a dietary aide when the CNA calls down for a substitute for lunch. Both staff members are under pressure: the CNA because the resident wants to eat with the other residents, and the food service worker because the trays must all get out in a timely manner.

So what happens? Most often, the CNA reports the problem to her charge nurse, who reports it to the unit manager, who reports it to the DON, who reports it to the director of dietary services, who speaks to the dietary aide. That is a lot of time spent and a lot of aggravation passed along, and it likely just leads to more tension between the CNA and the food service worker, which will spill over into the next call from the floor to the kitchen.

There are many other ways of handling conflict. Paul Hollings, a Massachusetts administrator, developed his policy after staff members in small discussion groups said they felt disrespected when another staff member reported a problem about them to the boss. Hollings knew that as adults his staff handled many difficult dynamics outside of work routinely. But most conflict policies in long-term care have an approach that takes the situation out of the directly affected staff member's hands, making the end decision one that no one is really attached to. Instead he developed and distributed the following policy:

> All staff will handle any conflict directly with the person with whom the conflict has arisen. This conversation is to be handled privately and in a calm manner. In the event that a problem is not resolved to the mutual satisfaction of both persons, it is acceptable to request the assistance of a supervisor or another person to help resolve the problem.
>
> The only exceptions to this understanding are for problems related

to abuse, breaking of the law, or other noncompliance issues that should be reported promptly according to policy.

The goals of this understanding are as follows:

- To address problems in a timely manner
- To avoid gossip
- To increase respect
- To increase trust
- To eliminate negative aspects of conflict
- To achieve positive outcomes to solutions
- To resolve conflict in a calm manner

In the aftermath of Hurricane Katrina, charge nurses and managers at homes in the New Orleans area had to manage unusual levels of conflict due to the stress of the situation. As one nurse explained it to us, many young CNAs no longer had the benefit of guidance from older family members after their families were displaced and separated, so she saw it as her responsibility to intercede when they got "hot-headed." She would take them aside, hear them out, calm them down, and help them see a way forward, helping them steer through volatile times. Her staff appreciated the help, demonstrating their loyalty to her in many ways as they settled down.

Loomis House in Massachusetts used a state workforce grant to provide training in communication and conflict resolution skills to every member of the staff, so anyone can call a quick caucus to resolve a conflict.

Understand and Adapt to Different Developmental Stages

Many middle-aged nursing home staff and supervisors lament what they see as a "lack of work ethic" in young CNAs. They see younger workers as caring more about partying and friends than about their work. They don't know how to relate to them and feel frustrated by what they see as people who are not as attentive to their work responsibilities as these older employees were when they were at this younger stage in their own lives. It is difficult to remember at forty what we were truly like at twenty.

The fact is that young people *are* different than their older counterparts. Developmentally, people are different at different ages. Different things are important at 20 than at 40. Brain scans show that the frontal lobe, the area of the brain that allows for judgment and executive function, isn't fully developed in most people until their mid- to late 20s. Until then, the part of the brain referred to as the brain's pleasure center is dominant. So next time you're tempted to shake your head at a 22-year-old and say, "What were you thinking?" remember that he or she may not have been thinking at all.

Geriatric psychiatrist Susan Wehry suggests that structure contributes to frontal brain lobe development. Supervisors help the young brain develop by providing structure in the work for young staff. By being explicit about what is involved in a task, breaking it into smaller steps, and checking in frequently, a supervisor can help younger workers stay on track. This will help them learn to plan ahead and see the consequences of their actions. Encouragement and positive feedback will foster their skills and sensitivities toward other workers.

Younger workers are also at a different stage of psychological development. According to Erik Erikson's theory on the eight stages of man, the developmental task of people in their 20s is to find intimacy and connection. Supervisors can motivate younger workers by recognizing their need for affiliation and recognition. All of us respond positively when we hear our name used, but it is especially important in working with this age group to use their names often and tune in to their abilities and unique attributes and interests.

In their book, *Managing Generation Y*, Carolyn Martin and Bruce Tulgan note that the perfect manager for this group is one who listens to their ideas, recognizes and mentors them, inspires them, and motivates them to excel at work. By valuing their contribution and recognizing their desire for further learning, we can help our younger staff succeed.

Young supervisors who supervise older staff members have their own dilemmas. It can be very challenging for a new, young nurse who is in charge of a unit with many older, seasoned CNAs to make changes. But a young, smart supervisor knows that she cannot do this work alone, and having CNAs she can trust and turn to is an advantage. Being honest about difficult dynamics can help turn this potentially difficult supervisory situation into one that benefits both. Simply acknowledging that the CNA has experience and is a valuable member of the team will go a long way in making this dynamic work out. Pairing up a new supervisor with an experienced nurse supervisor is also a good strategy for developing the supervisory skills of the new supervisor. A home that was investing in its nurses' leadership development had regular meetings among the nurses to talk about areas they found challenging. When some of the younger, newer nurses expressed their discomfort with exercising directive leadership, more experienced nurses offered explicit guidance on how to take matters in hand on the unit and keep the staff on task. The regular meetings among the nurses helped them turn to each other outside of the meetings. More experienced nurses checked in with their younger counterparts during the day and at shift hand-offs to encourage and support them in stepping into their supervisory role.

Help Staff from Different Cultures Understand One Another

Most U.S. nursing homes have workers from all over the world. This can lead to a rich variety of perspectives, but many American-born staff are reluctant to inquire about their immigrant co-workers' backgrounds. It is not unusual to hear administrators say that they have staff who were born in other countries but they're not sure which—"somewhere in Africa," they think, or "one of the islands."

Wide variations in cultural norms about death, illness, and ways of treating elders come into play in our nursing homes. Immigrants' struggles and challenges also affect their lives in ways that can spill over into work. Failing to discuss these things can hamper the relationship-building needed for residents' safety and quality of life.

Language barriers can further complicate matters. Residents find it hard to understand staff with accented English, and English-speaking American-born staff often mistakenly think they are being gossiped about when co-workers speak in their native languages in the break room or the hallway.

Body language also differs by culture. Looking someone in the eye, a sign of truthfulness in American culture, is a sign of disrespect in many other cultures. Yet we tend to assume we know what someone's body language indicates.

Clearly we need to talk about these differences, but immigrants who are striving to fit in may hesitate to ask questions about things they don't understand. So it is incumbent upon their supervisors to make sure that employees understand what is being communicated.

Farrell tackled this issue head on. He was on the job only two weeks when, during a meeting with the night shift staff, he told them how proud he was of the rich diversity among staff in the nursing home, as reflected in the 19 different first languages spoken by staff. He then added country of origin to each person's name tag to celebrate the diversity of the community, create conversation starters, and promote relationship-building. It worked.

Farrell borrowed the name tag idea from one of the major hotel chains, which has been doing it for years. This was the first time he tried it, and he was amazed at the positive effect it had. The name tags got people to ask each other questions, which helped them get to know and respect each other. He says he saw a kind of calm come over new hires from foreign countries when they saw their country of origin on a staff member's name badge, and theorizes that that immediate connection led to higher retention rates. He also saw that the tags allowed native-born staff to comfortably ask questions of foreign-born staff about countries many had never heard of.

Recognize Socioeconomic Differences—and Help Out Where You Can

The Long and Lescoe-Long study, *Identifying Behavior Change Intervention Points to Improve Staff Retention in Nursing Homes*, noted differences grounded in socioeconomic class that created conflict between CNAs and their nurse supervisors. These tensions, they found, cause a significant amount of turnover.

In the homes in the Long and Lescoe-Long study, most of the CNAs fell into the category of severe economic disadvantage. Yet most of the licensed nurses had a perspective shaped by their bootstrap experience, assuming that the CNAs had had the same opportunities they had had, and that they were more successful economically only because they worked harder.

The researchers also described organizational practices that created tension. CNAs had many people telling them what to do and few asking for their input, but nurses expressed frustration that CNAs didn't think more for themselves. The nurses ascribed that deficit to character flaws instead of seeing it as a product of the organizational environment—an environment that they themselves contributed to. For example, scope of practice requires that nurses do assessments so that when a CNA recognizes a problem the problem must still be verified by a nurse. It is frustrating for CNAs to know what they see and not have it count. And it is frustrating for nurses to be interrupted by CNAs coming to them to report problems for which the treatment is obvious. The system denigrates what CNAs know rather than honoring it.

Lack of empathy was a big factor in the negative dynamics, since the supervisors generally had no idea what the CNAs faced every day. That lack of understanding created its own cycle of distrust and misunderstandings.

Doing research the same year similar to Long and Lescoe-Long, Susan Eaton noted the loyalty that managers and supervisors engendered in low-turnover homes by showing empathy for the struggles of their CNAs. "In cases where administrators sometimes advanced people salary money if they needed a car or an emergency operation, workers stayed longer and felt more loyal," Eaton wrote. These supervisors knew that CNAs with problems are not problem CNAs, and they back up their empathy for the economic struggles of their staff with tangible help, as Farrell did when he referred a suspected drug user to his employee assistance program.

Lawrence Lindahl, an organizational development researcher, conducted research in the 1940s to study employee motivation. The studies were repeated with similar results in the 1980s and '90s. Time and again, the studies found, employees ranked high on their list a desire for employers to have a sympathetic understanding of their personal problems.

Going beyond a sympathetic understanding to providing real help will benefit both the affected employees and the nursing home. Many low-wage employees don't have access to traditional loans when they face a financial emergency, such as the need for a deposit on a new apartment or money for a car repair. Administrators who step in with loans, or set up formal emergency loan programs, report nearly 100% repayment rates and long-lasting loyalty from the employees they assist.

One administrator told us that learning about the barriers his CNAs overcame had given him a renewed appreciation for their dedication to the residents. "When they come in smiling, all wearing the same uniform, I just thought that everything was going well, but once I got to know each one individually, I came to realize that for some of them, just getting here on time took an unbelievable effort. Now I devote resources to help staff through tough times."

Don't Play Favorites

Few things are as toxic to the work environment as favoritism. If people think some co-workers get special treatment because they're friends of the boss, the organization has a serious problem. Usually, the people who are seen as favorites are the staff who managers appreciate because they make their work easier, being available when needed, pleasant to be around, and consistently good at their jobs. It is very easy for a supervisor to think: "They are making my job easier, so I'll do the same for them." Sometimes supervisors get into the rut of only seeing the staff they usually turn to. In this dynamic the quiet, more reserved but reliable staff can be overlooked. In one home-care agency the nurse managers were dismayed to learn that their star home-care worker was going to be leaving her job to move to another state because of her husband's employment there. They relied on her to mentor new workers and to take on the most difficult cases, and they appreciated her insight into the home situation and care needed. After the worker left her job, the agency invested in training four home-care workers to take on mentoring. What they found was that all four of the new mentors were equally as good and as reliable as the worker who had left. They had just not been seen because all of the positive attention had been focused on the one worker.

Another way managers can be perceived as playing favorites is when staff know that a co-worker isn't performing or has done something that deserves censure. If the situation is not resolved quickly, workers may assume that nothing is being done—or, worse, that the offender is a friend of someone important, so the infraction has been overlooked. If the worker was reported by a co-worker, it is important to let the person who made the accusation know that you are taking it seriously and investigating it, although of course you can't violate the employee's confidentiality by sharing the details of the investigation.

Micro-inequities are another, more subtle cause of ill will that can make people feel left out. These are small slights that may only be noticed by the person who feels slighted. A manager who avoids saying an employee's name because he can't pronounce it, but greets others in the group by name, is seen as slighting the employee not greeted by name.

Farrell tried to avoid committing micro-inequities by making sure he had personal contact with each employee through his rounds during the course of the week. By making a point of talking to everyone,

Farrell gave the quiet, reserved staff the chance to be known as well as the extroverts, and they all thrived under his leadership. By personally recognizing and relating to his staff through his positive personalized rounds, Farrell released endorphins that gave his staff a chemical boost.

Include Your Staff in Decision Making and Problem Solving

Team building has been a subject of research for many years. In his three decades of research, Lawrence Lindahl found that one of the top three things employees wanted from a job is "being in on things." A 2009 study[2] of nursing home staff confirmed the importance of being included in decision making and problem solving, finding that inclusive management practices led to higher retention rates. Study after study also shows that turnover rates among CNAs are significantly lower in homes where nurse supervisors listen, respond to CNAs' recommendations, and involve them in care planning.

Team problem solving helps shift the focus from shame-and-blame dynamics toward solutions. The more experience people have with thinking things through together, the better they'll get at it. Taking a quick caucus of the workers on a shift can be a good way of handling day-to-day problems as they come up. Bigger issues may require the involvement of people from all shifts and departments.

Including direct caregivers in care planning helps you make good decisions, enhance resident safety, and resolve problems. A basic tenet of quality improvement is that you need to know what your customer wants and needs, and the best way to find out is to ask your customers and those who work closest to them.

One of the New Orleans administrators we worked with after Katrina talked about how everyone had worked together during the crisis, pulling each other through by drawing on each other's abilities and ideas. That experience taught her how much frontline staff know, so she now includes them in all aspects of decision making. "When we are making a policy change or big decision, we'll invite the affected people in and say to them: 'If we do this, how will it affect you? What will be the result? Do you have a better idea?' Very often they'll have a better idea than what we had, because they know in a practical sense how it's going to work."

In another home, the DON pulled all the nurses together after the home received deficiencies for errors in administering medications and asked what had caused the problem. In the past, she had tried individually counseling nurses after receiving medication-related deficiencies, but the problems hadn't gone away. When she asked the nurses for their input, she learned about systemic problems that could be fixed. Interruptions were a big factor, so they came up with better ways to handle phone calls, CNAs' questions, and other interruptions to protect the charge nurses' concentration when they were giving residents their medications. Surprising to the DON was that her interruptions were also a factor. Counting medications takes concentration. In this open way of really looking at the root cause they also realized that the pharmacy was delivering medications at an inconvenient time of day, so they rescheduled the delivery time. By working together, the DON and her nurses finally—and permanently—resolved their medication-administration problems.

In another home, a proposed rearrangement of rooms to accommodate a new resident was met with dismay by the frontline staff, who knew it would not work for the residents involved. Sure enough, within hours the rooms had to be restored to their original arrangement.

Failing to ask for staff input can hurt your home as much as asking for input can help. When staff know that something that is being planned will not work and they aren't asked for their input, they lose trust in those in authority. They become disengaged and may start voicing negative sentiments.

Asking for input and then disregarding what people offer is worse than not asking in the first place. If you do that, expect staff to be silent next time you ask their opinion. If you decide on a different direction after asking for staff input, make sure to explain why you made that decision, and ask them if the issues they raised are satisfactorily addressed by the solution you chose.

Don't Blame Employees for Problems Caused by the System

Good supervisors take care not to blame employees for problems that are caused by the system. One DON was criticizing her nurses for failing to do some assessments when she realized that the problem was the strict limits the home had imposed on overtime. Since there were also several vacant positions on the nursing staff, there just wasn't enough time in the day for the remaining nurses to do everything. Instead of blaming her nurses for a human resources problem, she needed to concentrate on filling the vacancies.

As discussed earlier in this chapter, another common issue is the practice of CNAs hoarding linen, as they did in David Farrell's home. What this practice really signifies, as Farrell learned, is that the CNAs do not trust that they will have enough clean linen to do their job, so they stockpile what they will need in their residents' rooms. In other words, the "problem CNAs" in this scenario are actually people who care enough about their residents' needs to devise an end run around a flawed supply system. Maybe the solution lies in ordering more linens, rethinking the time and frequency of laundering them, or considering how and when to get the linens to the floor. One thing is for sure: A thousand write-ups will not solve the problem.

An employee who neglects to perform a basic duty or fails to follow official procedure may be raising a red flag. Before you blame or punish the individual involved, do a root cause analysis. Treat this like any other quality improvement process, investigating what is happening, getting input from your staff about what is needed, and pilot testing solutions.

A Tale of Two Nurses

At a nursing home that was stuck in a vicious cycle of turnover, absenteeism and contentiousness, nurses gathered to discuss how they were handling the stress on their shifts. One said, "I gather my staff in the morning and tell them 'We're like a bundle of sticks. If we work apart, each of us can be broken. If we stick together, we can't be broken. We've got to stick together to get the work done. And let's have fun doing it.' Then I pitch in and we get through the day." A nurse in the next unit over had a different approach. "I'm overwhelmed by what I have to do when we're working short," she said. "If I start doing the CNAs' job, I'll never get all my meds passed and my charting done. It's just too much. I just focus on my work and get as much done as I can."

As you might have guessed, CNAs loved working for the first nurse and did not like working for the second, who they perceived as thinking she was too good to get her hands dirty. The second nurse was young and didn't have much experience or any training in supervision.

She didn't realize how she was perceived by the CNAs, or how she was contributing to the stress that overwhelmed her. It had never even occurred to her that there was another way to do things until she listened to the first nurse.

When the DON realized how overwhelmed the second nurse was, she stepped in to help. She mentored her personally and started holding regular meetings for the nurses to solve workflow problems. The first nurse explained how she brought the staff together at the beginning of each shift and why it was so important to get the day off to a good start as a team. She talked about the benefits of pitching in, and how when she needed to step back to fulfill her other responsibilities, her staff protected her time. She talked about timing her work with residents so it coincided with the CNAs' work, in order for them to work together when CNAs needed an extra hand. She modeled teamwork and created an environment for teamwork among her staff.

The other nurses helped the second nurse problem-solve how to handle challenging issues of workflow. They talked through how she could change the timing of meal delivery to better match the pace on her unit. They also decided as a group to change the CNAs assigned to her unit, to make sure she had a strong, more cohesive team while she gained supervisory experience. With this peer support, the second nurse grew in her abilities and became a solid, effective supervisor.

Nursing homes seldom have the resources to provide supervisory training, but formal training is only one way to provide this important education. A more affordable option is to make supervisory training a part of your home's everyday operations through regular meetings among nurses about their supervisory responsibilities and by mentoring nurses to help them develop these skills. You can create systems that foster relationships, develop people's abilities, and involve people in working through problems together.

You can also help by asking your managerial staff about supervisory and workforce issues, just as you ask them about clinical issues. By focusing on this important aspect of their job, you are developing their skills, letting them know that good supervision is important to you and to your home, and modeling the people–development skills they need to help the rest of the nursing staff succeed.

When we decide that something is important we devote time to it. Good supervisory practices are no different. By helping our nurse managers and other department heads hone their supervisory skills, we lay the groundwork for better staff retention and resident outcomes.

Notes

1. In case you're wondering about the rest of them, Group 3 came in second. Apparently, having to rise to the occasion brings out good performance. Group 4 came in third, having let up on their efforts when they heard they were closer than they'd thought to the finish line.

2. Donoghue, C., and Castle, N. G. (2009). Leadership styles of nursing home administrators and their association with staff turnover. *The Gerontologist, 49,* 166–174.

## CHAPTER 5

Achieving Staff Stability

A Case Study*

The first step is that you have to be big enough to say what
you're doing isn't working. Then you can fix it, do it better and
move forward.

(Scott West, Administrator, Birchwood Terrace Healthcare)

THE FOLLOWING CASE STUDY demonstrates the use of a classic quality improvement process to achieve staff stability. Administrator Scott
West collected and analyzed the data, determined the root cause of the
instability in his home, developed specific interventions in response to
those root causes, and continued to tweak and measure his way back
to stability. We share this story because the problems at Birchwood
reflect practices throughout the field, and the solutions they used demonstrate what a difference management practices can make in achieving stability.

From 2004 through 2006, the three of us worked together to help
West and Birchwood Terrace Healthcare in Burlington, Vermont, im-
prove staff stability through a project that was funded by the Robert
Wood Johnson Foundation and The Atlantic Philanthropies. Called

---

* This chapter builds on content originally developed for and contained in the
Staff Stability Toolkit produced by Quality Partners of Rhode Island, available at
www.qualitypartnersri.org.

Better Jobs, Better Care (BJBC), the project was initiated with the premise that when jobs are stable and rewarding, then the care for residents improves. The project provided funding to coalitions in five states. BJBC in Vermont used some of the funding to work individually with nursing homes and other long-term care providers on organizational change efforts to become better places to work. BJBC–VT's steering committee sought out participation from leaders in the long-term care community, such as West who was President of the Vermont Health Care Association. He had worked previously at Birchwood Terrace and then had been gone for a period of time. When he returned, he immediately realized that there was too much instability. He was pitching in, plugging holes, letting staff know he appreciated them. And they were glad to have him back. He saw participation in the BJBC project as an opportunity to get help to stem the tide of turnover and absenteeism, and to stabilize his organization.

West was able to step back from the daily hectic pace and examine, in a deep and deliberate way, what kinds of behavior Birchwood was rewarding and how to change what it was doing in order to create a different result. It became the model for a major pilot program in which 254 homes across the country improved their staff stability through the same deep examination and resulting changes. That pilot, Improving the Nursing Home Culture (INHC), was funded by the Centers for Medicare and Medicaid Services and administered by Marguerite McLaughlin at Quality Partners of Rhode Island, the quality improvement organization where Farrell worked and for which Brady and Frank, as subcontractors, served as consultant faculty.

The practices at Birchwood were, and are, industry norms. Helping West and his team buck these norms and carve a new path to stability gave the three of us the opportunity to develop tools and practices to support his transformation that proved useful to the 254 homes in the INHC pilot, and to many others since. While Birchwood's experience of instability and prior attempts to address it were not unique, their ability to recognize that what they were doing wasn't working was. As part of a demonstration project, they set out on a new path with much better results. They used classic quality improvement practices to make sustained improvements, and their case offers a blueprint for change for homes across the country. Many of the lessons from Birchwood are reflected in this book in Chapter 2 on hiring and Chapter 3 on attendance.

The work at Birchwood Terrace became a model for Farrell after he left Quality Partners of Rhode Island to reenter the world of nursing home administration. He used many of the Birchwood Terrace interventions and tools as he looked to make improvements in the nursing homes he was involved with.

Background

At the time we worked with Birchwood Terrace, it was a Medicare- and Medicaid-certified nursing facility owned by Kindred Nursing Centers East, LLC, a subsidiary of Kindred Healthcare, Inc. Birchwood was licensed for 160 residents and employed 186 people. It had a sub-acute unit, a dementia unit, and a regular long-term unit. It was pretty similar to most homes across the country in its basic structure, resident population, and care and services.

The group overseeing BJBC–VT identified Birchwood as a prime site for on-site support because of its leaders, Scott West, the administrator, and Sue Fortin, director of nursing. Both were actively engaged with colleagues in their state who recognized them as leaders in their field. BJBC–VT knew that West and Fortin would make good use of on-site assistance, and would share their lessons openly for the benefit of others.

When Birchwood began its participation in BJBC–VT, it had lost 92 licensed nursing assistants (LNAs) (Vermont's equivalent of certified nursing assistants) in the previous 12-month period, and 28 nurses during that same time. On our first visit, we met West as we walked up to the front door. He was washing the windows because he was short staffed in housekeeping. We could sense the strain among staff. Everyone was working hard and running fast to keep up. We noted the brag board was empty, the staff break room was uncomfortable, and no one had signed up for the employee appreciation event. We used three days of focus groups to talk with almost everyone on staff and began to see how their efforts to respond to the day-to-day crises were often perpetuating and exacerbating the problems.

We helped West and Fortin collect and analyze financial and human resource data, and they saw the evidence: their crisis-response practices, despite being the standard in the field, were creating negative incentives. They redirected their resources and immediately started to stabilize. They worked next to improve their supervisory and management practices. By spending smarter and supervising better, they cut their turnover by two thirds. At the three-year conclusion of the project, they had a waiting list for licensed nurses and only two open LNA positions.

Using Qualitative Data

At the start of our on-site work, we gathered information from staff about their day-to-day experience. We talked with groups of staff on all shifts, units, and departments during two weekdays and one Saturday. The staff described the stress they felt as they worked short more often than not, and often had co-workers who were new or unfamiliar with what was needed. Too tired after working a double shift or after the stress of working with tired or temporary co-workers, they would make a last-minute call the next morning that they weren't coming in. People described the strain they felt, their worry for residents, and their own exhaustion.

Staff described newly hired staff who didn't know what to do or who quit before the end of the first day. No one had time to show them around or patience for their questions or mistakes. With so many leaving so quickly, it was hard to tune in to anyone new. The expectation was that the new employees wouldn't last, so current staff just hunkered down and took care of their own assignments.

These long-time staff were hanging in but felt hurt that their loyalty wasn't being appreciated. They'd gotten what felt like scant raises and meanwhile saw the home offering financial incentives to new people being hired. Each time they saw a newspaper ad from Birchwood offering a sign-on bonus or starting wages that put earnings for brand new LNAs on par with what they were making with their years of experience, they felt resentful and unappreciated.

Some staff asked why people who came in as a last-minute substitute got $5.00 more an hour than they did for the same work. We met a number of employees who indicated that they had gone from full time to per diem so they could get the extra $5.00 an hour. The move also allowed them more distance from the stress. Some shifted to full-time work elsewhere, just picking up extra shifts at Birchwood as they could because the hourly rate for last-minute assignments was so much better than the regular rate.

Nurses and LNAs with regular schedules and assignments often found themselves working with different co-workers each day, including someone newly hired, someone from an agency, and often someone who was working a double or other extended hours. Supervisors were feeling extremely stressed, some to the point of tears. The stress was causing conflict and interfering with teamwork. Just as Susan Eaton mapped out in her "vicious cycle," the stress on staff was causing more last-minute absences, so the remaining staff worked short, making their work all the more stressful. As a result, some staff quit, others switched to per diem, and too many didn't come in for their shift because they were worn out.

We discussed these issues with West and suggested he consider redirecting his bonuses to reward good attendance instead of rewarding people for taking last-minute assignments. He was initially taken aback. He asked a common question: why should he reward people for doing what they are supposed to do? We talked about how the current system was inadvertently rewarding the opposite. His staff got paid better when they took the last-minute assignments than when they came to work as scheduled. Some of his staff were responding to the current reward system in ways that eroded his full-time roster, by calling off tired after having picked up a shift for the higher pay, or coming in to work exhausted from working too many shifts, or switching off the regular schedule and just working per diem. His incentives weren't serving the interests of continuity and stability as much as rewarding reliability would.

Another source of information as West was getting to the root causes of his instability was the company's annual employee opinion survey. It mirrored the information from the focus groups, revealing that a large number of staff felt a high degree of stress. They expressed this in response to questions about whether management cared about them as a person, whether there was good teamwork, whether the management team was making a good effort to get replacements when employees were absent, and in a key indicator, whether staff would recommend their workplace to others. Many staff also expressed a high level of concern about poor communication, lack of support, working short, lack of supplies, and favoritism. Many respondents said Birchwood was not a welcoming place for new staff.

A key factor in the management team's ability to see staff's experience clearly was that the responses to the survey were tabulated for three groups: department heads, licensed staff (nurses), and non-licensed staff (LNAs, food service, and housekeeping staff). This allowed management to see how differently these three groups of staff experienced the workplace. The differences were striking. While department heads were aware that there were serious problems due to turnover and were dealing with the daily crises as best they could, the survey results indicated just how seriously the stress was affecting staff and that, in fact, the management team had different perceptions than the rest of the staff about the depth and nature of the problems.

Managers were trying to provide support, promote morale, and plug the holes in ways many good leaders do in similar situations. West was hands-on—passing trays, making beds, transporting residents. Staff appreciated his attempts, but they still felt overwhelmed. Pizza parties and other attempts to improve employee morale were unsuccessful because they weren't alleviating the stress the staff was experiencing.

Even as department heads were working diligently to address the problems, they were unaware of just how depleted and demoralized their staff were, especially their nurses. It is not unusual for people to have different perceptions based on their different positions within an organization. Managers thought communication, teamwork, support when working short, and overall morale had improved. The survey information gave them a clear, although somewhat demoralizing, picture of what they were actually dealing with. In some categories, like the ones detailed in Table 5.1, the perceptions of different groups appeared to be polar opposites. They particularly took notice of the fact that nurses had the lowest morale.

The level of negative responses was shocking to the management team because of how hard they were working in the face of the daily stress, and how much they knew they did care about their staff. It is not uncommon for satisfaction surveys to provide responses that are surprising, and even disappointing, to the management team.

Birchwood's management team took a deep breath and let the hurt pass so that the information could be used constructively. They realized that it was better to know how people were feeling than not to know, and that if their efforts to support people weren't being felt, that it wasn't an indication that they didn't care, but it was an indication that their caring efforts weren't working. They determined to do something different so that their caring would be felt.

Information from employee satisfaction surveys is like seeing the tip of an iceberg. While you know you are seeing a part of something, you also know that you have to look deeper to see it all. This can be difficult because if there is information that does not look good at the surface, you may be fearful of what you will find if you look more

Table 5.1. Variations in Group Perceptions

When employees are absent, there is a strong effort to get replacements.

	Strongly Agree (%)	Agree (%)	Neither Agree nor Disagree (%)	Disagree (%)	Strongly Disagree (%)
Department heads	29	57	14	0	0
Licensed nurses	14	36	14	29	7
Hourly staff	17	17	17	17	33

Teamwork in my department is good.

	Strongly Agree (%)	Agree (%)	Neither Agree nor Disagree (%)	Disagree (%)	Strongly Disagree (%)
Department heads	57	43	0	0	0
Licensed nurses	13	13	27	20	27
Hourly staff	33	33	0	0	33

Management cares about me as a person.

	Strongly Agree (%)	Agree (%)	Neither Agree nor Disagree (%)	Disagree (%)	Strongly Disagree (%)
Department heads	43	57	0	0	0
Licensed nurses	7	13	27	13	40
Hourly staff	17	50	0	0	33

I would recommend this to a friend as a good place to work.

	Strongly Agree (%)	Agree (%)	Neither Agree nor Disagree (%)	Disagree (%)	Strongly Disagree (%)
Department heads	43	43	14	0	0
Licensed nurses	20	13	20	27	20
Hourly staff	33	17	0	17	33

closely. But when there is a problem, only by facing it, and understanding its full dimensions and causes, can you make the necessary changes to get to a different outcome.

A survey can indicate areas of concern, but it doesn't get to the root cause of the concerns. To find out what is causing the concern, and therefore what can be done to fix it, leaders need to dig deeper. Often focus groups are a useful way to learn more about the nature of staff's concerns. At Birchwood, the focus group discussions that had occurred prior to the satisfaction survey pointed to a number of practices that were leading to the problems employees were expressing.

These practices were efforts on Birchwood's part to stem the tide of instability. The practices were standard in the field, but they weren't working. In fact, they were making things worse, accelerating the instability, and generating hard feelings among the reliable staff who were the core of the facility's care team. Crisis practices that made things worse included the following:

- *Not taking the time to hire right:* Like many homes experiencing turnover, the need to fill the vacancy felt so immediate that they rushed the hiring process to get people on board. Feeling an urgent need to fill vacant spots, they brought on new people they might not have hired had they felt less pressured. They didn't realize that taking chances with people who weren't working out was causing more stress to their regular staff than if they had been more selective and brought someone on who would be able to make an immediate positive contribution to the team effort. Having so many new staff not work out made the current staff less welcoming to new staff, because they had low expectations and no reserve energy to invest in helping someone make it or getting to know someone who likely wouldn't. This contributed to new employees feeling poorly welcomed, having difficulty settling in to the job, and leaving.

- *Inconsistent assignments for new staff:* Because the need for workers was so great, new staff did not get time to settle in or get the benefit of a serious orientation. New staff were often given different assignments each day, plugging that day's hole, which meant they couldn't get to know their co-workers, residents, or supervisors. One day they were working on the Alzheimer's wing, another day in subacute. The differences in the pace, routines, and residents' needs made it feel like a new workplace every day. Often they were filling in where there was already instability, which meant that there wasn't enough continuity among the day's co-workers to provide new employees with the guidance and assistance they needed. As a result, many new staff left immediately, feeding the cycle.

- *Piecemeal hiring:* Desperate to fill the schedule, they lost control of it, accepting whatever times a potential new employee was willing to work. Fortin said that she couldn't get nurses to work full time (almost every nurse who interviewed insisted on a per diem or part-time spot). Making piecemeal arrangements as they could to bring people on board, they then had more part-time needs without having solid full-time schedules to offer to other new employees. With new staff coming on only for certain days and shifts, the schedule was a daily jigsaw puzzle, in which schedulers scrambled to fill holes and fit people in as they could.

- *Sign-on bonuses:* To be competitive with the other homes in the area, and to attract applicants, Birchwood offered sign-on bonuses to new employees in nursing. This was upsetting to current staff, who felt undervalued by comparison. In addition, it drew in people based on a cash incentive, not a caring incentive. And given the instability in the workplace, some of these new employees hung in there long enough to collect their bonuses, and then they were gone. This added insult to injury for long-time staff.

- *Last-minute assignment bonus:* Birchwood offered a bonus of $5 an hour for certified nursing assistants (CNAs) and $10 an hour for licensed nurses to cover for staff who called in absent at the last minute. This too was a common practice in the area. It skewed incentives so that it was a better deal financially to take a last-minute assignment than to work a scheduled shift, leaving dependable staff feeling short-changed by their reliability. It also created the sense that people could always call off, because the home would make an arrangement to get someone in, and also that if someone did call off, they could always pick up another shift later in the week, for more money, rendering the schedule almost meaningless. Staff had very little cohesiveness because people did not have regular teams to work with. Supervisors felt the stress of having to make out an assignment list each day once they were able to take stock of who was there. For residents, there was little continuity in daily caregiving. While money is not the primary motivator for people working in long-term care, when the job becomes highly stressful, money becomes a greater factor in direct correlation with the degree to which they feel dissatisfied with the other factors that motivate them. This bonus system contributed to staff disengagement and the take-up rate on it reflected the shift away from a commitment to full-time work and daily continuity.

- *Baylors:* In another scheduling deal, Birchwood used a common practice known as a "Baylor" program, through which staff who worked two 12-hour shifts got paid as if they had worked for 30 hours. While this had originally been instituted at Birchwood to allow full-time staff to have more weekends off, the program had taken on a life of its own, expanding to weekday use. Staff working the Baylor shifts described how exhausted they were by the end of their second day, and that they often needed a couple of days just to recover. They plodded through but their exhaustion diminished their helpfulness and made them an added stress for co-workers to work with. They often weren't available to attend any educational sessions or organizational meetings on days they weren't scheduled, either because they were so tired or because they had taken other jobs during the open days that the Baylor arrangement created. They had little continuity with residents, staff, families, or clinical care from one work period to the next.

Individually these practices were typical responses to staffing needs, used by homes all across the country. Collectively, they each contributed to an erosion of stability, feeding Eaton's vicious cycle.

While we had a sense, based on the focus groups and employee satisfaction survey, that these practices were at the root of staff's low morale, undermining management's efforts to boost the staff, we needed to go a step further to see just how much of an impact these practices were having and therefore what to do about it. We designed a "drill-down" process through which West and Fortin could collect quantitative data documenting what we were hearing in the focus groups about the erosion of their core group of full-time staff, the steady loss of newly hired staff, and the costly unintended implications of their financial incentives.

Using Quantitative Data

Data is crucial to decision-making. Data moves a leader from having a sense of something to knowing concretely what is happening and therefore being able to make decisions about what to do. The conventional industry interventions Birchwood was using to address common industry problems needed the scrutiny of data collection and root cause analysis. West often used data collection for quality improvement (QI) in clinical areas and so it made sense to him to use data, root cause analysis, and a QI process to tackle his workforce challenges.

To get concrete about how Birchwood's own practices might be contributing to employee concerns, we formulated data collection tools to allow West and Fortin to identify links between the home's financial incentives and its staff instability. These "drill-down" tools were subsequently used by the 254 nursing homes in the Quality Partners pilot, and then refined further as part of the Quality Partners Staff Stability Toolkit. A sampling of these tools can be seen in Appendixes A and B, and they are available electronically at www.qualitypartnersri.org (accessed through the HATCh workforce tab).

The tools capture basic information in two areas: the current employment situation and impact of the current financial incentives. To analyze the current employment situation, we structured the tools in response to what we heard from the focus groups about the erosion of the base of full-time employees, the high rate of turnover among newly hired staff, the loss of longevity particularly among supervisory staff, and the early exits of staff who had sought employment based on the sign-on bonuses. Because the employees' status and longevity seemed so deeply connected to the incentives created by the last-minute assignment bonus and the sign-on bonus, we structured the analysis of the financial incentives to capture the cost of these practices compared to what was being spent for practices that would incentivize stability.

While it took time to collect the initial data, once the process was in place, West was able to continue to track these areas as he formulated alternative interventions, and therefore to see how well his interventions were working. The areas for data collection were such important markers for stability that they were areas that continuously needed to be monitored.

Looking at the Current Employment Situation

Composition of the Current Staff: For a snapshot of the current employment situation, the tools looked at the composition of the current staff. How many nurses and LNAs were working full-time, part-time, per diem or Baylor? Given the piecemeal hiring and the Baylor arrangement, the incentives favored non-full-time work. How much were staff shifting in that direction? Did that have any bearing on the degree to which nurses were burned out or staff felt contention and stress? This data gave Birchwood a way to look at the current situation in terms of what positions they needed to fill, why they had holes in their schedule, and the impact of hiring for either full-time or part-time work. They found that they had shrunk their full-time nursing staff. Their nursing staff was made up almost entirely of part-timers or Baylors.

Employment by Length of Service: Next, the tool collected data on staff in terms of length of employment to see how many staff were relatively new and how many had been there for some time. The tool allows the user to have an overview of who is employed by their longevity along a continuum that spans from employment of less than six months through employment of more than 10 years. Every home has groups of staff who have been with them a long time, some who have a shorter tenure, and others who are relatively new. Generally, it is to an organization's benefit to have the long-time staff as the biggest block of employees because these staff are loyal to the home and knowledgeable about residents and about processes of care. Looking at percentages of staff that fall into different length of service categories allowed West and Fortin to see that they were experiencing a significant erosion among their "steady Eddies." This was a big red flag for them.

Terminations by length of service: The tools took a step further in looking at terminations by length of service. West could see how long people had been on the job before leaving in categories from one month or less, to two or more years. While West and Fortin had known that a significant number of new employees weren't lasting, it was shocking for them to see just how many didn't make it. It confirmed what staff had said in focus groups and in the employee survey, that the work environment wasn't conducive to settling in new employees. In the Quality Partners pilot, this also turned out to be an eye-opening source of information, as a number of participating homes were astonished by how quickly new employees were leaving. When those pilot homes calculated how much they spent in money and effort to hire a new employee only to see so many not make it, it was a call to action to make improvements in the hiring and welcoming processes.

Another red flag for Birchwood was the number of employees who left after they collected their sign-on bonus, an indicator that the bonus was contributing to instability by drawing people attracted by the money who did not stay, either because of the caliber of person being hired or the stress of the work environment they were hired into.

The tool also divided terminations by employee or employer choice. Seeing how many people left by employer choice let them know their hiring practices needed to be improved. Bringing someone on board without proper screening was contributing to costly instability.

Turnover replacement costs: The drill-down tool next gave West a way to calculate just how much this turnover was costing Birchwood. He was able to analyze both individual and annual organization-wide costs for turnover. Together we identified costs that occur in replacing an individual LNA, nurse, or other staff. Costs included recruiting and hiring, staffing the vacancy, training, and orientation expenses. Looking at the expense of losing just one employee put a concrete dollar amount on efforts to stem the tide of turnover. While West had access to information about industry average costs for turnover, it was eye-opening to look at his own home's specific costs. The total annual cost of turnover was staggering.

Looking at the Financial Incentives

Financial Incentives: The drill-down tool listed all the financial incentives currently in use. West was able to collect data on how much he was spending on areas his staff had raised as concerns as well as other areas that seemed to be contributing to instability. How much was he spending on bonuses paid for last-minute assignments, compared to any spending he was doing to reward good attendance and reliability? What was the cost of shift and weekend differentials and higher per diem wages? What was the hourly rate for Baylor payments when calculated for the number of hours actually worked? How much was he spending on sign-on bonuses compared with raises, longevity bonuses, or refer-a-friend bonuses? While West and Fortin had been aware that these practices were costly, it took seeing the data to realize just how much these incentives were costing Birchwood annually. Coupling the financial costs of these practices with the results in stress and instability gave West and Fortin a clear look at what was happening, why, and what they could do about it.

Analyzing the Data in Detail

West collected the data in May–June 2005 and we analyzed it together in June. When we looked at the composition of his current staff by employment status, it was immediately clear that full-time employees made up the lowest percentage of staff, particularly in supervisory and

Table 5.2. Composition of Current Staff (June 2005)

Position	Full Time	Part Time	Per Diem	Baylor
RN Total: 30	8 27%	4 13%	14 47%	4 13%
LPN Total: 27	15 55.5%	0 0%	5 18.5%	7 26%
CNA Total: 77	37 48%	8 10%	7 9%	25 32%

management positions. Of 57 licensed staff, only 23 (less than 50%) were full time (Table 5.2).

The data showed a link between the high percentage of non-full-time supervisory staff and the organization's instability. Nineteen nurses out of 57 worked per diem, without consistent enough schedules to be able to maintain continuity in care to residents and management of staff. Of 30 RNs, responsible for consistent leadership of the nursing team, only 8 worked full time.

The other number that jumped out in looking at the composition of the staff was that a third of the LNAs and a quarter of the LPNs were Baylors, working their two 12-hour shifts and being paid for 30 hours. While in theory this looked like it might work, the reality was that working two 12-hour shifts left many people worn out and not at full capacity to carry their share of work. Many who worked Baylor also worked another job and were running on empty.

For West and Fortin, the data placed in stark relief an explanation of what they had been experiencing. Working only a few shifts a week, per diem and Baylor nurses weren't available to follow up on resident or staff issues or to participate in facility initiatives. This explained problems in leadership, morale, and communication. CNAs had different supervisors each day, each with their own way of doing things, their own expectations of the staff, and, in many cases, limits on the degree to which they engaged with the teamwork and communication issues on the floor.

West and Fortin saw that there were not enough people providing leadership and oversight. They looked person by person at who had made the switch from full time to per diem, and knew that many were long-time employees who had been the backbone of the organization. The ranks of the full-time staff were eroding. They were compounding the imbalance by their hiring of people into part-time and per diem rather than full-time positions. They were indeed in a vicious cycle.

They knew immediately that they had to get control of the schedule. To have daily stability, they needed to get back to having primarily full-time positions and some part-time employees with guaranteed set schedules who could be counted on. They realized that neither Baylor nor per diem arrangements contributed to continuity. Looking at the financial incentive data (Table 5.3), they saw that Baylors were getting paid the most, and then per diem staff who worked last-minute assignments.

West and Fortin conducted an analysis in which they looked at everyone's rate of pay. For the Baylor and per diem, they factored their incentive pay into their hourly rate. What they saw "blew [their] minds!" *Birchwood was rewarding the behavior it was trying to stop and not rewarding the behavior it sought to encourage.* This was a radical realization. The best deal in the house was to work as a Baylor. Birchwood, like many other homes that use Baylor systems, was paying its staff for hours they didn't work. How could they afford to pay people when they weren't there? As a result of the incentive pay, Baylor nurses made more per hour than the director of nursing, with far less responsibility.

The next best deal was to work per diem and take a last-minute assignment. By contrast, there was no financial benefit to working full time and committing to a schedule that the facility could count on. There was no bonus for having perfect attendance. They saw that they had lost control of the schedule because staff had converted from full time to per diem and Baylor and were picking up last-minute assignments when it fit into their individual schedule to work. By accommodating each person's schedule in order to keep them, Birchwood was losing the steadiness and consistency needed to provide a good work environment. Even in its hiring process, they had been hiring per diem if that is what people wanted, tipping the balance even further into this vicious cycle.

Table 5.3. Financial Incentives—Bonuses (June 2005)

Bonus	Extra Per Hour	Annual
Baylor	Work two 12s, paid for 30 hours	$268,944
Per diem	$1 add-on to regular hourly wage	$51,012
Last-minute assignment	RN, LPN: $10 CNA: $5	$360,000
Perfect attendance	$0	$0

We reflected back on West's earlier question: Why should he reward people for doing what they were supposed to do? Now the data provided conclusive evidence and he realized that the opposite was true—under the current system, the full-time dependable staff were the least rewarded. West and Fortin knew immediately that they needed to win their employees back from per diem to full-time and shift resources to favor dependability.

He knew that more full-time positions would contribute to a stable environment for new staff, which would help stem the tide of turnover. He also needed to figure out who was leaving and why. The data on current staff by length of service and terminations by length of service were disturbing (Tables 5.4 and 5.5). The length of service data compounded the staff composition data. It showed that many nurses in charge were new (60% of RNs and 52% of LPNs had been there less than a year). There was greater stability among LNAs than among nurses, which meant that LNAs frequently experienced the disruption of new supervisors with new systems. While a few long-time staff members were hanging on, the numbers reflected a precipitous decline in longevity.

Knowing how much staff stability depends on having the largest percentage of employees be long-time core staff and the smallest be new staff, West and Fortin were dismayed by the numbers. At Birchwood, the smallest percentage of staff was the long-time core staff. Among the nurses, the largest percentage had been there less than a year and were in positions that were frequently turning over.

So, who was leaving and when were they leaving? Of 66 CNAs who had left in the past two years, 15 had left within their first month of employment, and another 19 had left within the first three months. This was a clear indication that something was not working well in the hiring process or in the orientation. It was compounded by the piecemeal composition of staff, leaving little structure or continuity for helping new staff settle in. Placing new employees in an unstable environment was a set-up for failure.

Among the nurses, another factor emerged. While some nurses were leaving within the first few months, the bulk of the departures were occurring at or just after the six-month mark, just after the payout of their sign-on bonus.

Because Birchwood Terrace needed to replace so many staff, they were doing what all of the homes in the Burlington area were doing: paying sign-on bonuses. It turns out that they had paid out $50,000 for

Table 5.4. Current Staff by Length of Service (June 2005)

Position	< 6 mos. (%)	6 mos.-1 yr. (%)	1-2 yrs. (%)	> 2 yrs. (%)
RN	10	50	20	20
LPN	11	41	33	15
CNA	12	14	68	6

Table 5.5. Terminations by Length of Service (June 2005)

Position	1 day–1 mo. (%)	1-3 mos. (%)	3-6 mos. (%)	6 mos.–1 yr. (%)	1-2 yrs. (%)	> 2 yrs. (%)
RN	18	18	18	27	18	0
LPN	7	13	33	27	20	0
CNA	23	30	23	16	3	5

sign-on bonuses. The data were striking in drawing the correlation at the 6-month mark between the sign-on bonus kicking in and the high rate of turnover of licensed nurses (Table 5.6). It was apparent that some employees were leaving at the 6-month mark as soon as they collected their bonus. The unwelcoming environment provided no incentive to stay any longer. Here was an expenditure that was clearly not contributing to stability.

By contrast, Birchwood was spending very little on refer-a-friend bonuses because staff weren't referring their friends. And, just as the current system did not reward dependability, it also did not reward longevity. There was no bonus for longevity and the 2% raises did not amount to nearly as much per individual as people receiving the sign-on bonus got.

West and Fortin saw that they were spending a lot on practices that contributed to instability. How much was their turnover costing them? Using a tool designed to add up the cost of screening, hiring, and training a new employee and covering for the vacant position,

Table 5.6. Financial Incentives—Bonuses (June 2005)

Bonus	Amount Offered	Quarter Paid—Annual Estimate
Sign-on bonus paid after 6 months	RN: $2,000 LPN: $500 CNA: $250	$12,500–$50,000
Referral bonus paid after 6 months	RN, LPN: $1,000 CNA: $500	$1,500–$6,000
Longevity	$0	$0
Raises	Average 2%	$90,710

Birchwood was able to calculate the turnover cost per position. Its annual total cost for turnover for all positions was $453,940. Birchwood had not previously calculated its turnover costs, and they turned out to be alarming (Table 5.7).

Birchwood was *spending more than $1 million per year on turnover* and practices that accelerated the turnover. By contrast, it was spending *one tenth of that amount on investments in stability*. In fact, the only investments the home was making in stability were a 2% annual raise and a modest referral bonus program (Table 5.8).

As soon as West and Fortin saw the data, they understood why they were getting the results they were getting. When asked later to share their lessons learned, they harkened back to the day they saw the data. They said they knew they had problems, but it was only when they looked at the data that they really understood what was happening and what they needed to do about it.

The Plan for Change

While West and Fortin had known that their problems were serious, they had been so caught up in each day's crisis that they had been unable to step back and recognize that their crisis responses were only fueling their problems. The data was both shocking and grounding. It helped them see how serious their situation was and how urgently they needed to act. And it helped them know exactly what they needed to do.

Table 5.7. Turnover Costs (Calculated in June 2005)

Position	Per Person	Annual Cost
RN	$4,899	$53,889
LPN	$4,193	$62,895
CNA	$3,207	$205,248
Other	$2,692	$131,908
Total 2004		**$453,940**

Table 5.8. Instability versus Stability (June 2005)

Costs of Instability	Investments in Stability
Last-minute bonus: $360,000	Perfect attendance: $0
Baylors: $268,994	Raises at 2%: $90,710
Sign-on bonuses: $50,000	Referral bonuses: $6,000
Turnover costs: $453,940	Longevity bonus: $0
Total: $1,132,934	**Total: $96,710**

They realized that what they were doing wasn't working and that they needed a new approach. They focused on three goals for a six-month effort (from July 1 to December 31, 2005) to stabilize staffing:

- Increase the percentage of full-time staff

- Increase the percentage of newly hired staff who stay

- Improve attendance.

Goal 1: Increase the Percentage of Full-Time Staff

To increase the percentage of full-time staff, West worked with his corporation's district office on a new wage package that made working full time more attractive. West was able to free up resources to do so by eliminating the last-minute assignment bonus and phasing out the Baylor program. By having the data to show his corporation how he was going to spend differently he was able to make the case for higher wages. He was able to show why his current incentives weren't working and how he could stabilize quickly by changing those incentives. He had wanted to give raises but because his staffing costs had been so high, he hadn't been able to do so before. Now, he was able to redirect the resources that had been inducing instability into a wage increase that only staff who committed to a regular schedule were eligible to receive (Table 5.9).

West and Fortin then began an aggressive internal marketing campaign. They sat down one-on-one with each part-time, per diem, and Baylor staff member to talk about what the raise plus benefits would mean for them and to tell the staff that they were phasing out most of the per diem and Baylor positions. They explained their goal to restore stability and talked about how important it was to them to have staff who worked consistently and could give continuity of care. They talked about the importance of stability for teamwork and quality care. They knew this was not just a financial equation for employees and that they had to win back people's trust that Birchwood would once again be a good place to work.

Table 5.9. Raises for Staff Committing to a Regular Schedule (August 2005)

Position	Old Wage Range	New Wage Range	Raise Amount
CNA	$9.25–$10.50	$11.50–$12.75	+ $2.25
LPN	$15.00–$16.70	$18.00–$20.50	+ $3.00–$3.80
RN	$18.00–$20.50	$23.50–$26.00	+ $5.50

By December 2005, they had gone from 60 full-time employees in the nursing department to 80. Several staff members converted from per diem back to full or part time. Many former employees returned. As Birchwood brought on new staff, it almost exclusively hired for full-time positions. Very quickly, a positive cycle had started. As the environment stabilized, more new staff stayed, more former full-time staff converted back to full-time, and even more former staff, who had left at the height of the instability, returned. By December 2006, they had 96 full-time employees in nursing, an increase of more than 50%.

The shift was largely cost-neutral; dollars that had gone to Baylors for hours they didn't work were now going to full-time employees for hours worked. Birchwood spent more on health insurance costs as they had a greater number of employees who converted to full time and took up the benefit. Yet, they saw this additional cost as an investment in stability, compared to the instability caused by how they had been spending before.

Goal 2: Increase the Percentage of New Employees Who Stay

There were two dynamics to the wage bump that West and Fortin had to deal with. First, they anticipated that the advantage of the wage increase would be short-lived, and that their competitors in the area would quickly move to match their wages. Second, they hadn't been prepared for the number of applicants that the wage bump attracted. Until their competitors raised wages to catch up with their new wage levels, Birchwood attracted a large pool of applicants drawn by the comparatively higher wages, not all of whom were well suited for work at Birchwood. After a few false starts with quick terminations of new employees, they revamped their screening and hiring process. Making good hiring decisions was a key element of their strategy for their second goal, to increase the percentage of new employees who stayed.

Increasing retention of new employees involved both a better hiring process and a better welcoming process. When West and Fortin examined their current hiring process, they realized they needed improvements on several levels. Looking at the data on terminations by employer choice, it was clear to them that Birchwood had been hiring people who wouldn't have made it through a better screening process. We worked with the management team to identify steps they could take to ensure that someone they decided to offer a job to would be a good contributor to the Birchwood team. West told the department heads and managers that putting together a good team was their first priority. He wanted his department heads and nurse managers to do their own hiring and take responsibility for building their teams.

Hiring Skills

A number of department heads asked for help, explaining that they didn't know how to go about interviewing or checking references. The maintenance director spoke up, asking where to begin. So we asked him to articulate what he most needed from someone working for him. The head of maintenance easily listed off a number of needs: besides basic competence, he needed the person to have good common sense and be able to juggle a variety of demands with good skills in prioritizing, time management, and handling all the personalities of the people needing help. We asked him what would be a typical scenario someone working for him would face and he described one. We suggested that he present that scenario to applicants and ask how they would handle it. That put his mind at ease so well that other members of the management team began developing their own scenarios.

Through training sessions like these with department heads, managers learned to focus on character traits and explored ways of using the screening process to determine who would be a good fit. Managers did mock interviews with each other posing as applicants. Those posing as applicants played out particular scenarios or personalities that they had run into in the past, so managers had practice handling difficult situations—how to draw someone out in the interview process to get an idea about their interpersonal abilities. The managers looked through applications of people they had hired who had not worked out and discussed potential red flags. For example, they reviewed an applicant whose previous work history was one of steady work and demonstrated reliability—but she had not worked out at Birchwood. When they looked carefully at her work history they saw that her work had involved a lot of sitting. Working on her feet in a fast-paced environment didn't work for her.

Screening System

West and Fortin decided to focus their recruitment on new entries to the field whose approach to the work could be influenced through a training class. They preferred to hire through their own training class rather than draw people who had worked at other facilities in the area and perhaps not performed satisfactorily. The process of getting into the class became the point for screening. To get the right people into the class, they set up a three-part process, each requiring attendance and timeliness as one of the screens. First was the open house that included an information session and a tour of the building. Each manager took two or three applicants on the tour, invited questions, and encouraged them to interact with residents. Applicants were told this was their chance to convince the manager to have them back for an interview. While applicants were getting to see the building, managers got to see the applicants' abilities to relate to residents.

After the tours, the managers met together to decide which applicants to interview. They made three piles—yes, no, and maybe. They reviewed the applications, looking for red flags. They identified areas to be probed in the interviews or reference check. By doing this as a group, managers helped each other figure out what to look for and how to shape the interview. They were sounding boards for each other as they all developed their ability to make good hiring decisions. Applicants had two more appointments to keep: the interview and a pre-employment physical. If the applicants made it to the class, Birchwood found that they would make it through the class and onto the floor. By making the screening at the front end of the class, they retained everyone they trained.

Having the training class as the stepping-stone to employment also gave Birchwood a chance to make a better welcoming process, starting in the classroom. The instructor served as a bridge, helping managers and class members figure out the best fit for new assignments. As the class was concluding, the instructor was able to introduce new employees to their future supervisors and co-workers.

Welcoming System

Birchwood worked equally hard to revamp its welcome so new employees would settle in well after the class was over. West and Fortin campaigned for a better welcome just as they had for the conversion back to full-time schedules. They talked to everyone about the goal of stability and the importance of helping good new people stay. They explained the steps they had taken to improve the screening process, so that now current employees could have trust in the strong likelihood that any new co-worker would be a good addition to the team. They asked everyone's help in bringing new employees on board.

Because the evening shift was the hardest to stabilize, they piloted a better welcoming process there. The evening shift supervisor was exceptionally good at his job. He set an example that the rest of the building then followed. On his shift the entire staff took responsibility for helping new co-workers succeed. The experienced staff members worked one-on-one with the new staff and took new staff with them on breaks and to meals. Sometimes the staff members had pizza together to welcome their new workmates. Rather than isolating the support for new employees to one staff member appointed to be a "mentor," all current staff took responsibility for supporting new employees in addition to the specialized support provided by the official mentors.

New staff members had a two-day orientation. On day two, a nurse in charge of the mentor program set up each new employee's schedule, taught the person how to read it, and connected the new employee with a mentor. The classroom instructor and the leader of the mentor program followed up with the new employee daily throughout the first few weeks. Managers and supervisors made it a priority to check how new staff were doing, the first day and onward. The management team discussed new staff members individually at their morning stand-up meeting and kept track of their progress as they settled in. Since they had all discussed the person's hire, they were all eager to know how each person was working out. When someone didn't work out, they dissected the potential reasons why: Was it a hiring mistake, a problem in the welcome, or some other reason it wasn't a good fit? What could they learn about it so they would do better next time? If there had been any questions about someone hired, managers wanted to know how those questions panned out. They were all invested in making good decisions that built a strong, solid team.

In June 2005, 34 of the 66 CNAs who had left in the previous 12 months had left within their first 3 months of employment. By December 2006, almost all of the new employees were staying through the first 6 months and beyond.

Reflecting back on the change in practice, Fortin remembers their desperation to plug a hole in the schedule, even when it meant hiring someone who had been "no call/no show" at another facility. "We'd hire them and hope they'd work out," she said. As they adopted high standards in their hiring, they stopped hiring people they had doubts about. As they started hiring better, staff welcomed the new hires better, and they stayed.

It caught West and Fortin by surprise how much the staff supported them in the more careful hiring process. Their reliable staff members wanted management to hire reliable staff. As staff trusted the quality of the people coming on board, they felt the investment in helping them settle in was worth it. And as staff were more welcoming to new co-workers, newly hired staff were now set up for success.

Goal 3: Improve Attendance

Birchwood began to embrace high standards for attendance as well. Farrell helped West work with the scheduler to develop ways for her to track employee attendance. They developed an organized system for handling last-minute absences and documenting them. The managers saw that with three or four call-offs every day in June 2005, they were constantly focused on that day's staffing. Managers, the scheduler, and supervisors had been so busy plugging holes and pitching in that they hadn't had a way to figure out how to get their heads above water. With a system now for capturing absences, they could get a handle on it. Managers received the information for every employee in their department. Employees received their monthly attendance record with their paycheck.

At regular manager meetings, the attendance was reviewed by individual and by department. West made it a focus at the meetings to discuss unscheduled absences so that, as a team, they kept as close a watch on attendance as they did on census. West, being a firm believer in process improvement, told his managers, "What you collect is what's important to you. When we focus on something, we make it work." Managers analyzed the absences for patterns and met one-on-one with each individual with significant absences to communicate their concern. Rather than a strictly punitive approach, managers worked with employees with a lot of absences to reduce their hours to a more manageable schedule or make other adjustments in their assignment to help them succeed. They terminated staff who couldn't be depended on despite these interventions.

West and the managers made it a priority to focus on supporting attendance. As they were out there pitching in, they talked about not wanting anyone to be working without a full team of people scheduled to work, because that added stress and made it harder to give good care. They stressed good attendance in their hiring process, and mentors and supervisors emphasized it as well.

Reflecting back on the question of rewarding staff for being able to be depended on to do their job, they instituted perfect attendance bonuses that staff accumulated month by month over a year. Employees who worked all their scheduled hours in a given month got a $25 bonus credit for that month. At the end of the year, all the bonus credits were paid out, so that the bonus also rewarded longevity. The maximum payment was $25 for each month of perfect attendance, or $300 for the year. It felt good to staff to get a pat on the back for their reliability, after having felt resentful when others were getting paid more to come in at the last minute. In a positive cycle, the more people had good attendance, the easier it became to come to work. The stress diminished. Working with a full staff made the work much more manageable and created an atmosphere in which people worked well together.

From Stability to Cohesion—Building Skills and Systems

Within just a few months, by the fall of 2005, Birchwood was already feeling the positive effects of its stabilization efforts. As they began to stop the vicious cycle of turnover and absenteeism, West and Fortin knew that a key element in getting a positive cycle going would be leadership among the ranks of their managers and supervisors. They asked the managers and supervisors to take on their leadership roles in a more deliberate way. Supervisors who had been caught up in the vicious cycle of instability, just trying to hold a shift together, now needed support to lead under new circumstances, in a way that fostered better teamwork. Supervisors struggled over how to hold people to a high standard without being harsh about it. Many voiced their unease in not knowing how to handle challenging situations with their staff.

So West began focusing on management skills with his department heads and with Birchwood's nursing management and supervisors. At morning stand-up, in addition to looking at any clinical and operational issues that needed attention, they included workforce issues. It started with looking at attendance and how well new employees were working out. It grew into teachable moments where managers helped each other think about how to handle staff-related issues.

West and Fortin began having regular meetings with nurse managers focused on workforce and workflow. Nurses explored ways of being neither lenient nor harsh, but instead holding their staff to high expectations and helping them meet those expectations.

The nurses began to problem-solve together and become a support group to each other, with Fortin playing a key role in facilitating
the process. Staff brainstormed ways around problems each was facing.
In their collaborative problem solving on work*force* issues, one nurse
discussed a new employee on the subacute unit who wasn't keeping up.
Another nurse volunteered to have the new person switched to the
slower pace of her unit. In problem solving on work*flow* issues, a nurse
talked about the morning stress. She said sometimes she cried when
she saw the breakfast cart come because the staff didn't have the residents ready for their breakfast. Fortin said she would talk with the food
service director about holding the trays for that unit until they were
ready to receive them. Another nurse offered to have the cart come to
her floor first.

In the newly stabilized work environment, the nurses talked about
other areas where they could benefit from making adjustments to take
the flow of work in hand. Nurses from different shifts met together
at these meetings and were able to shift some responsibilities in ways
that better distributed the work. As they made these adjustments, they
contributed to reducing stress and further stabilizing the work environment. The positive cycle continued to gain momentum.

Within a fairly short period of time, the nurse managers were
able to start to look at ways to individualize care for residents and take
charge of workflow. They started to identify changes that would allow
them to take into account residents' individual preferences for waking
and sleeping times. This led to a very thoughtful discussion the nurses
had about the medication pass. They talked about residents who would
be good candidates for review and potential reduction in medications,
and also how to time some of the medications so that staff didn't have
to wake up residents just to give them a medication. The medication
pass created a hectic morning for residents and staff. They made a plan
for working with physicians and the pharmacist to do a careful review.
Excited by nurses' creative brainstorming and concrete solutions, West
wrote a congratulatory note to all who had participated:

> We had a great meeting with the people from Better Jobs Better Care
> Grant. Everyone brought insight and the reality of what we do. Hon-
> est discussion is what will move us forward and improves our system
> of delivering care for our residents and staff. . . . I am impressed and
> thankful that we recognize that sometimes our systems are set up be-
> cause "it is just the way that we have always done it." Let's break the
> mold, think outside the box, and make it happen!

Birchwood was experiencing a new energy. Staff members were able to shine. They were working together better and finding new ways forward.

The Results

By the following May (2006), Birchwood had created a new norm—daily stability. It had broken the vicious cycle. It had seen a 33% increase in full-time staff. With high retention and attendance, it was fully staffed each day, so care became manageable and the environment more positive and supportive. West continued working with department heads to grow their leadership skills. He said, "I expect more from them, and I'm working with them to meet my expectations." Fortin said she had learned that "leadership is all about relationships. Anyone can be a leader. You have to understand your impact and bring out the best in the staff." She was supporting a number of her nurses in pursuing further education.

West and Fortin noted positive differences in the year since their data analysis:

- Now that we have more staff, people aren't as stressed. They are more able to help each other out. We don't hear "not my hall."

- Nurse managers model teamwork instead of conflict.

- We have trust among the team; we can say "time out, let's look at this."

- Now we are hiring for full-time positions, and we take the time to hire right.

- The schedule runs smoothly now—no favoritism—and now we have consistent attendance.

- Consistent attendance is allowing us to move to consistent assignments.

- There is better team problem solving on the units.

- Now we can take on individualized care.

Each positive development provided grounding for the next. Because they had accurately addressed the root causes of their instability through a multi-dimensional approach, they were able to continually improve, and to sustain their improvements over time. Bringing new

Table 5.10. Workers Who Left (2004–2005 compared to 2006–2007)

Workers Who Left	2/15/04–2/15/05	2/15/06–2/15/07
LNAs	92	30
RNs	18	3
LPNs	10	6

Table 5.11. Gains in Full-Time Staff (2005–2007)

	2/15/05	2/15/07
Open CNA positions	14	2
Open staff nursing positions	6	0
Full-time CNA	31	51
Full-time nurses	18	31
Per diem employees	22	6

employees into a stable environment had helped them to stay, and the stability was also having an impact on long-time employees. Staff were now staying (Table 5.10).

Not only were people staying in employment, but they were also coming to work according to their assigned schedule. Attendance continued to improve. In December 2006, Birchwood paid out $13,000 in attendance bonuses. Most of the employees had been able to get at least one month's worth of a bonus, and so the bonuses were a real boost when they came at the end of that year. Everyone celebrated on the occasion of their being given out because West and Fortin stressed to them that by their good attendance, they had made a better work and care environment for everyone.

While the $13,000 payout seemed like a large expenditure, it was small in contrast to the $360,000 they had paid out in bonuses in the previous year for people to pick up last-minute assignments to cover for others who were absent. Not only was it a bargain; it was also a wise investment. Having seen how demoralizing it had been for his steady staff to watch others get paid so much more for so much less commitment, West knew now how important it was to let staff know, in monetary terms, how much he valued their dependability.

## PART III

Moving
the
Flywheel

## CHAPTER 6

The *How* of Change

IT IS NOT JUST *WHAT* YOU DO but *how* you do it. The How of Change is a change model developed by B&F Consulting, in partnership with Quality Partners of Rhode Island. The model uses both the science and the psychology of change. The *science* of change involves basic quality improvement practices: data collection; root cause analysis; cause-specific interventions; small pilot tests; evaluation; midcourse adjustments; and then collaborative spread.

The *psychology* of change focuses on the *how* of the change process. For any change process to be successful, all those involved in and affected by it need to be involved in identifying problems and solutions. The psychology of change builds on the intrinsic motivation of employees to do a good job, starts where people are, builds their capacity for critical thinking and collective effort, and creates a climate for honest discussion about what is working and what is not.

Both the science and the psychology of change require skills in critical thinking and collaborative action. Both require strong interpersonal relationships that allow for the true give-and-take necessary to look objectively at what is happening and what is needed. In the How of Change, the focus is on systems change—an intense process of exploration by the people involved, to solve the problems they face so they can give the best care possible. This approach uses quality improvement and organizational development tools for organizational growth and improvement.

When an organization takes on something new, leaders have to be willing to accept some failures and learn from mistakes. Rather than having individuals bear the blame for what doesn't work, a systems approach analyzes where systems did not work and how they can be improved so they do. Leaders need to create an environment for honest debriefs and analyses, where staff can talk openly about what they see as impediments so these concerns can be addressed. Taking the time up front and then along the way to recognize and address barriers improves chances of success in any endeavor.

The core lesson of the How of Change is that it is not just *what* you do, but *how* you do it.

In this chapter, we discuss the following:

- The *why* of change

- The *how* of change, in terms of the science and psychology of a change process

- The *how* of high involvement

- Putting it all together: the *how* of change.

The Why of Change

Change is a fact of life. In long-term care change is constant and inevitable.

Whether you've been in long-term care for decades or just recently entered the field, you've seen changes. Certainly, if you think back to the first time you ever went to a nursing home, you know the changes since then have been significant, and mostly for the better. As the field of long-term care has evolved with new knowledge and new oversight, many changes have clearly been beneficial, while others have felt hard to manage. There have been many changes in how nursing homes are paid and surveyed. With continual growth in knowledge about good care and workplace practices, there have been gradual changes in standards of practice, industry norms, and public expectations. Today's nursing homes have more competition and fewer resources, while caring for residents with greater frailty and more complex needs.

How leaders take on these changes really does matter. How you manage and operate day to day affects how successfully you can handle changes that come your way and how you can initiate changes to improve your organization's performance. Instituting changes to support and involve staff provides the foundation for continued improvement and gives your organization the lift it needs to respond to externally driven changes such as changes in regulations or payment.

Reflecting on her experience during Katrina, one New Orleans nursing home administrator said,

> If you ever have to have an evacuation or you have to go through something to this extent, I hope that you have your daily business in check because, if you don't, you will probably fail. If your employees don't know their roles, if they don't know the communication system, if they don't have faith in you, if they don't value you, then you probably lost before you ever really get started.

While implementing a new government or corporate mandate is not on the same scale as a challenge of Katrina's magnitude, your ability to succeed at any endeavor depends on the changes you can make so that your staff know their roles and you have systems to support staff to perform at their best. Being steady and stable today makes you ready for whatever tomorrow may bring.

Instability is stressful and saps energy and resources that could otherwise be spent on making improvements. If you are in the midst of Eaton's *vicious cycle of instability*, it can be hard to find the time to step back and look at ways to intercede to break the cycle. However, if you don't, then the steady flow of government and corporate mandates will feel insurmountable. Changes in management practices to support and develop your staff are a necessity to be able to break the cycle. Through simple changes, you can shift from putting out fires to working together to prevent them. Functioning more effectively gives you the footing to initiate positive changes and to handle whatever comes your way.

Staff stability is the prerequisite for better quality of care and more satisfied staff, residents, and families. When your staff, residents and families feel good about the care you provide, the word gets out. You become the place where people want to come for care, and the place where people want to work. Better census brings in the resources to improve some more. Like the flywheel effect referenced by Jim Collins in *Good to Great*, this process generates a positive cycle.

The How of Change: The Science and Psychology of Change

The Science of Change

The "science" of quality improvement involves basic steps:

1. Collect data to develop an accurate picture of the current situation.

2. Analyze the root cause to determine why it is happening as it is.

3. Pilot test interventions specifically designed to address the root cause, to figure out on a small scale what will work and what will be needed for it to work organization-wide.

4. Remeasure to determine whether the intervention is working and whether there are any negative effects that need to be mitigated.

5. Adjust the intervention, because change is an ongoing process that benefits from continual checking and tweaking.

6. Spread effective practices through an inclusive process that allows for adaptations to fit different circumstances in different areas of the organization.

Collect the Data

West and Fortin at Birchwood (Chapter 5) knew they had problems with instability. It was only when they collected the data that they were able to see the nature and extent of their problems and begin to determine the root causes. Seeing the data was their "aha" moment. Quantifying a problem allows you to hone in on it and address it. One unionized home in Connecticut didn't have problems with turnover because union jobs had such good benefits that staff didn't easily leave them. However, the home had daily instability from unplanned absences. Staff complained bitterly about working short-staffed. The administrator knew that he scheduled enough staff every day but that on many occasions it was staff absences that led to working short. When he collected a month's worth of data on unscheduled absences, he was astounded to see just how frequent they were. He tabulated the costs of these absences in overtime and saw immediately a source of his home's financial difficulties. He took the information out to his staff and offered bonuses to individuals for perfect attendance and to teams of staff for the most shifts worked without a call-off. He tracked the results publicly and everyone was able to see that the improved work environment they experienced was directly related to their improved attendance.

Conduct Root Cause Analysis

Don't play pin the tail on the donkey when you're trying to address a problem. Going at it blindly makes it strictly a matter of luck if you succeed. Root cause analysis is a process for determining *why* you are getting the results you are getting. Note that it is equally important to conduct a root cause analysis of your successes as it is your problems. Root cause analysis helps you know what you need to do to address a problem, and it also lets you know why you were successful when you succeed, so that you can sustain that success over the long term.

Nursing home leadership teams conducted root cause analysis by using *discovery assignments* to learn about the causes of their instability as part of their participation in Quality Partners of Rhode Island's 2004–2005 CMS Pilot on Workforce Retention, an arm of Improving the Nursing Home Culture. To learn more about turnover among new employees, members of the homes' leadership teams interviewed staff who had been there less than a year, asking them what it was like to come in new and what would have been helpful to do to welcome new staff. They asked what would have helped the new staff members to have a better experience. While the data showed how many employees left within the first month of employment and thus identified it as an area to address, the discovery process helped explain *why* people were leaving, so that interventions could be targeted accordingly.

One home participating in a 2010–2011 Advancing Excellence project promoting stability in inner city nursing homes learned through a similar process that the staff who had been asked to serve as mentors felt frustrated by the lack of support they received from upper management and were themselves on the verge of throwing in the towel. In response to being asked about their stresses, staff said that when they intervene to address problems they see with new employees, they are not backed up by their supervisors and thus they are ignored by the staff they are being asked to mentor. They've soured on being mentors. While the home thought it had a viable program in place to stabilize employment among newly hired staff, the leaders learned that not only were they continuing to lose these new employees, but also they were vulnerable to losing their long-term dependable staff who were stressed by the position the mentorship program put them in.

Pilot Test

It is always better to start small so that you can learn as you go and make the necessary adjustments on a small scale before taking a new approach organization-wide. Pilot testing allows you to see what is possible and opens up new possibilities that might not be apparent under current operations.

In pilot testing, start where you have the best chance of success, with a group of people who work well together and are open and eager to try something new. Start in a way that relieves burdens rather than adding to the work. Look for building blocks that can get you traction. Think of the game Pick-Up Sticks. When you drop all the sticks on the table, they fall in such a way that some are clumped together in a pile in the middle and others are more on the periphery, not entangled. You have more success in the game when you pick up the pieces on the periphery first, and then work your way slowly toward the more challenging pieces. As you carefully remove one stick after another, the knotty pile becomes less challenging. Finally, the last stick, that originally was buried, now stands alone and is easy to pick up.

At a large urban nursing home that was moving to a new physical plant from a very old building, staff's sense of what was possible had been shaped by the limitations of their current environment. The living space in the old building had very little privacy for residents. In the new environment, residents would have private and semiprivate rooms. "Lights out" at 9:00 p.m. had been the common practice in the large multi-person rooms. In the morning, as soon as the first people stirred, everyone was awakened by the noise. Having people go to bed and wake up by their own natural rhythms seemed impossible in the old environment. Residents had given up their own routines, and staff couldn't conceive of how to manage what they thought would be chaos in the new environment if people got up of their own accord.

Through pilot tests they explored new ways of organizing services that currently ran on their institutional clock. Each unit undertook a small experiment. One worked with the kitchen on making food available more flexibly during the morning hours. Another worked with activities to support activity and engagement during a wider range of hours, more flexibly scheduled and individually focused. Doctors, dietitians, nurses, and certified nursing assistants (CNAs) worked together to pilot test liberalizing diets among a small group of residents for whom it would be easy to make changes. Doctors, the pharmacist, and nurses did a spring cleaning in which they individualized the medication pass. While it had seemed overwhelming to change embedded routines, making "bite-sized" changes helped staff see what they could do. They worked together to tweak the changes and then shared what they had learned with others throughout their organization. Pilot testing allowed them to make small changes on an experimental basis where they could keep the learning and the process manageable.

Remeasure

As you pilot test, keep track of the impact. You'll want to see if your changes have a positive impact, and to monitor potential negative effects. Review the data together and discuss what to do about it. As one home in Massachusetts was eliminating its use of alarms, a team of CNAs, nurses, housekeeping, and other unit staff met daily with nurse managers to look at falls, agitation levels, how needs were being met, and the impact on staff. The first week, they stopped use of alarms only during the day shift. At the end of the week, as a group they decided they could proceed to the evening shift, and then the following week, they completed the removal of the alarms on all three shifts. By meeting as a team each day to look at the impact, everyone was able to see the positive results and discuss strategies to mitigate any emerging problems. Staff then had confidence in the approach. Because they could see the benefits and had the assurance of help with the problems, they were comfortable to proceed.

Make Adjustments

Nothing ever goes according to plan. A common mistake in the change process is to put all the time into crafting the change up front and then roll it out, thinking the work is done. A pilot test is just that—a test. By testing on a small scale, you can learn what works and what doesn't and make the necessary adjustments. Even rocket scientists have to make adjustments. The trip to the moon involved thousands of adjustments as scientists at NASA tweaked the trajectory a little to the left, and a little to the right, to achieve a smooth landing. To guide a change successfully, have mechanisms in place to be able to monitor and check in and make midcourse adjustments.

A home in Massachusetts that pilot tested *gentle awakenings*, through which residents awakened according to their own timing, hoped that the change would result in improvements for residents and staff. But staff worried that some residents might experience hunger going so long between dinner and a later breakfast. So they monitored residents' weights during the transition. Sure enough, a few residents were losing weight. They were able to beef up their late night food offerings and address the problem. They also documented improvements in residents' mood, decreases in use of anti-anxiety medications, and less stress for staff during that busy morning time. By measuring and remeasuring, they could see the benefits and make the necessary adjustments to address the problems they encountered.

As staff put change in place, you will want to keep in close contact with residents and staff who are affected by the change. The home that removed alarms attributed its success to its process of bringing staff and management together each day. Staff and management reviewed what had happened, what issues had come up, and what adjustments they needed to make.

Making adjustments is a key part of the change process. No change can be figured out entirely in advance. As we move forward with a change, we learn about ways we need to tweak our efforts. If something in your original plan is not working, talk with people about what other possibilities there are. Talk about unexpected issues that come up. Every change causes unintended side effects. We need to address those as we go along.

Some people think that you put a change in place and you're done. In fact, this is an iterative process. Expect that this will need your attention throughout the period of change and focus on the change process until the new practice becomes the new norm.

Spread

Every group has early adapters, people who wait and see, and those who are the last to join in. Early adapters are open to change and can roll with the ups and downs in traveling uncharted territory. People who wait and see can jump in to change when they see how it works and that there are benefits to it. Those who are the last to join in will come along when the tipping point has been reached and the new way of doing things replaces the old way.

Your early adapters are your champions of change. They can teach others how to make it work. At the large urban nursing home that tested changes in preparation for its move to a new building, staff on each unit volunteered to share their experiences with their small tests of change with their colleagues on other units. They were both compelling and concrete. They had seen the benefits of the change and could explain how residents blossomed far better than management could have explained the ideas in theory. And they were able to provide the concrete information about how to make it work because they had lived it. Their enthusiasm made them terrific ambassadors, and their experience made them valuable resources to their co-workers.

Many organizations that transition to consistent assignment start with the unit and shift with the most willingness to take it on and the best chance of success. Once those staff are able to report how consistent assignments actually make their day easier because they can anticipate their residents' needs and organize their time accordingly, other staff are more willing to take it on. Staff share common fears, such as being "stuck" with hard-to-care-for residents. Knowing that these fears are effectively addressed gives other staff the assurances they need to go forward.

Operating under two systems is one of the hardest parts of the change process. As the new practice takes hold, it becomes a relief to eliminate the old system and go building-wide with a change. When Maine General at Glenridge in Augusta instituted gentle awakening on one unit, the food service staff worked very closely with the charge nurse and CNAs to figure out how to schedule meal delivery in time as each person woke up. Their old tray line didn't work for this unit, so they found themselves operating a tray line for most of the building and delivering trays as needed for the one unit. As staff saw the benefits of having residents well rested when they ate their meals, another unit expressed interest in moving to gentle awakening. At that point, the food service staff asked that they shift entirely to the new system rather than operate two different ways. They had already developed a new way of operating the meal service that enabled staff to provide breakfast for residents as they awakened. Having worked out the process, they were eager to apply it to all the units. By spreading the change in morning wake-up times, they were able to align their entire kitchen operations with the new practice on all the units. As the dietary staff learned how to decentralize food service in the morning, they were able to extend the decentralization to other meals and to snack times. Now, when residents are up late at night and want a sandwich or a bowl of soup, they can have it because the food service staff spread what they learned to all shifts and all times.

After you have successfully piloted the change and it is the new norm, then spread it throughout your building. A benefit of pilot testing is that it may ease staff resistance. Resistance is often grounded in worry about how something will work. By pilot testing, other units have an opportunity to watch the process unfold and see the benefits. Then, instead of being worried, they are able to look forward to the change because they've heard the positive results from the pilot area.

The Psychology of Change

It is not just *what* you do, but *how* you do it. A memo from the administrator or director of nursing (DON) will not work as well as an inclusive group process. Effective change starts with good relationships. Stephen R. Covey wrote that quality, the *result*, is a function of quality, the *process*. He describes a people paradigm: "You cannot continuously improve interdependent systems and processes until you progressively perfect interdependent, interpersonal relationships."

In quality improvement (QI), using only the science of QI isn't enough. For QI to be effective, leaders must engage staff in figuring out how to implement these QI practices and in identifying organizational impediments that need to be addressed. We call this the "psychology" of change.

The Improving the Nursing Home Culture Pilot used a holistic approach to quality improvement that took into account both quality of life and quality of care factors, engaged staff in the change process, and addressed true root causes of change. At the end of the project nursing home leaders from across the country met to compare notes on what had been the keys to their success. Hands-down, leaders said that *changing the way they made changes* is what made the difference. They learned how to involve their staff in the change process, and this ensured that their changes were meaningful and effective.

The Psychology of Change has key components:

- Build on staff's intrinsic motivation.

- Personalize by asking, "What would you need in this situation?"

- Start where people are and build from there.

- Build people's capacity for change through small successful steps that get the flywheel moving and serve as building blocks to the next change.

- Use "experiential" learning so that people see, through their experience, the why of a change.

- Create an environment where people feel free to speak up, even if what they are going to say is not what the group is looking to hear. As Jim Collins says, you have to "create a climate where the truth can be heard."

Build on Staff's Intrinsic Motivation

As Susan Eaton wrote in "What a difference management makes!", "Good care could be its own reward." She quoted a nurse who said, "When people speak who haven't spoken for months, or when I see a light in their eyes that hasn't been there for ages, it makes it all worthwhile." In every home she studied, Eaton noted the consistent CNA response to the question, What do you like about the job? "I enjoy helping people, helping the residents, giving them support, keeping their spirits up, making them happy."

The enduring caring with which nursing home staff approach their job was demonstrated during the Katrina crisis. One DON, speaking about her staff's courage and caring during those scary days, told us:

> Crisis doesn't build character. It reveals character. We are watching on TV and they're seeing their entire city flooded to the rooftops, not knowing if their husbands are okay, if their children are okay. But they hung in there and they cared for these individuals.

At the large urban nursing home that was engaging in a major change, staff members involved in testing changes said that, to succeed, they needed to know the change they were making would make life better for residents. As that home transitioned from rotating to consistent assignments, staff who had initially resisted because they feared they would be "stuck" with hard-to-care-for residents watched with relief and joy as they were able to turn around difficult situations by getting to know each resident better. When Salvietti rolled out her new approach to absenteeism at community meetings (Chapter 3), she started by saying she wanted to make sure that there was enough staffing every day so that residents could get the care they needed, and staff could work without being shorthanded. When the home in Massachusetts worked to take off alarms, their first step was to explain to staff how alarms actually did more harm than good, so that staff understood that what they were doing was worth doing.

As you take on any change, be transparent about why you are doing it. Explain the benefits to residents. That is what motivates staff. If it is a change that results in better care for residents, they will support it.

Personalize

To personalize, we have to put ourselves in the place of the resident or staff member and consider how we ourselves would respond to a situation. When we look at a care practice change we need to understand that our residents are not different from us. In fact our residents *are* us, only older and frailer, and in need of care. If the current way that care is provided is something that we would have a hard time tolerating, then we should assume that our residents will have a hard time with it too.

Personalizing the experience, asking ourselves if we would want to live here, gives us insight into what needs to be changed. One of the best examples of someone who personalized the experience in order to understand what needed to change is Joanne Rader. Years ago, as she was starting to understand that the bathing experience was not pleasurable for residents at her nursing home, she asked her staff to bathe her. Her experience of being bathed by her staff gave her the direct experience that enabled her to understand what needed to change. And what the experience was like on the receiving end of it. This led to her seminal work in changing bathing practices in nursing homes around the country, captured in a book and video called *Bathing Without a Battle*. This work is so valuable that in December 2003, the Centers for Medicare and Medicaid Services (CMS) sent a copy of the video to every nursing home in the country. If you can't find your copy, you can order one at www.bathingwithoutabattle.unc.edu.

Putting ourselves in someone else's place in a very direct way gives us insights that guide and inform the work to individualize care. Since Joanne's work, we've heard from administrators who've spent the night in nursing homes. Being bathed and spending the night in the nursing home where you work are quite major experiences; you may be a bit overwhelmed at the prospect and feel unable to take something like this on. We have some suggestions for personalizing the experience in smaller doses:

- Sit in a shower chair and experience being wheeled down the hall in a Johnny.

- Wear a chair or bed alarm, or, if you still use restraints, sit with one on for 30 minutes.

- Lie in a resident's bed with your eyes closed and your senses attuned to the sounds and smells, the feel of the sheets.

- Take a shower in the shower room.

- Eat a meal.

It is important to put yourself in the resident's place and ask yourself, "How would I feel about this if I were in this position?"

The best way for staff to understand the benefits to residents of a change you are considering is to have staff ask themselves what they would need if they were in this situation. If you are thinking of taking off alarms, have staff wear an alarm for 30 minutes. If you are considering changes in the nighttime routine, ask staff what they would need for a good night's sleep. This builds on staff's intrinsic motivation to make life better for residents by helping them put themselves in a resident's place and see what they would need if they were living at their nursing home.

Start Where People Are

Have discussions with your residents and with your staff about what they are experiencing. Leaders in homes participating in the CMS Improving the Nursing Home Culture pilot asked residents what they needed for a good night's sleep, what their morning routine had been, and other questions about their daily life experience. At the large urban home, leaders asked residents what it was like on the first day after staff rotated assignments and leaders were taken aback to hear how much rotating assignments negatively affected residents.

Create a space of safety where your staff can raise questions and concerns and have an open dialogue, so that together you can sort out what is working and what is not. Staff and residents might be worried that what is working well now may be endangered by a change. You'll want to hear from them directly about what they experience, about which things to keep and which things to change.

When we listen to what staff and residents have to say about their experience, we learn what is working and what is not. This guides us in our change work.

One Connecticut home was eager to transform its bathing areas into "spas." When we met with CNAs, nurses, and housekeeping staff in each of the work areas, we learned that many aspects of the current bathing environment weren't working for the staff. Several of the bathing areas leaked in ways that left the floor wet and difficult for safely transferring residents. The doors were situated in ways that made it hard to provide privacy for residents. The lighting was inadequate. Before they could have confidence in a move to spas, staff needed to know that their current problems would truly be addressed. Starting where the staff was, with a need to fix the leaks, enabled staff to have confidence that other changes to remodel the space would mean that residents could have more dignified and private bathing experiences. Starting where people are builds trust and allows change to occur in sequential stages.

Build People's Capacity for Change

Each positive experience of change builds staff's capacity to take on the next one. So, too, each positive change opens the door to new possibilities. Once again, it is not just *what* you do but *how* you do it that matters. Often, in a change process, an organization anoints a committee to work on an issue, and that group mirrors the noninclusive process usually used in the organization, making decisions based on their own best judgment without engaging everyone on staff in thinking through the situation. Instead, use your change process to build people's capacity for change and tap into the wider wisdom of the staff as a whole. By widening the inclusion, you ensure that you have everyone's best thinking, and you build a wider rank of people who can be involved in future efforts.

At Maine General at Glenridge in Augusta, Connie McDonald, the administrator, wanted to take on culture change. Through focus groups, we learned from staff that it really pained them to come into a resident's room expecting to see someone only to find out the resident had died and someone else was now in their bed. They had to gather themselves together in the midst of their responsibilities to the new resident.

McDonald invited staff to join a committee to work on better ways to handle how deaths occurred in their home. In their first committee meeting, members reflected on their own customs related to death in their own cultures. Then they talked about what worked well and what didn't work well in their nursing home. Finally, they had a memorial service in which they were each invited to talk about residents who had passed away over the years.

Committee members then conducted similar discussions throughout their organization, with every department, unit, and shift. They learned a tremendous amount about what currently worked and didn't work and solicited ideas from staff about how to improve the experience. They enlisted volunteers for various ideas and talked through with their co-workers ways to make sure the ideas worked. For example, they decided to set up a special board by the time clock where information could be posted when someone died so that staff could learn about it when they clocked in, instead of when they came up on the unit. Such an idea would depend on everyone using it, so it was essential that everyone believed in it. Night shift staff, for example, had to see the value of coming down to the time clock to post the news after someone died so the next shift would have time to compose themselves. When we debriefed about what they had learned from the experience, staff said that it worked because the change was something that mattered to them, and their input had shaped the change. Everyone contributed and everyone benefited. They all learned how to engage in an effective change process and then were able to take on new challenges to continue to change their culture.

Often staff hesitate to become involved in a change process because they doubt their opinions will count. Managers hesitate to turn responsibilities over to staff because they fear staff will not take into account everything that needs to be considered. In this case, McDonald, the administrator laid out clear parameters—such as not lighting candles in memorials, due to fire safety. They also laid out clear permissions, giving staff the green light to proceed with the purchase of items for a comfort cart that would help families sitting vigil during a loved one's dying process.

When St. Camillus Health Center in Massachusetts was looking to make more use of its van for residents to go on outings, the administrator, Bill Graves, and DON, Sandy Godfrey, set up a process for staff to discuss their ideas before they proceeded with scheduling outings. A criterion was to make sure that there were enough staff on hand to help with residents' needs and enough staff remaining in the building to care for those residents who stayed behind. Staff had the opportunity to use their critical thinking and problem-solving skills, and the confidence to know that they could go forward with their plans because they had considered all the key factors. Their positive experience with changing the use of the van led them to further creativity in providing in-house activities as well.

Most staff are good problem solvers in their own lives, and when the door is opened for them to use their problem-solving skills at work, they do so very well. Each experience of change builds their capacity to take on the next change.

By starting small, staff can see more possibilities. At the large urban home, CNAs and activities staff pilot tested individualized activities with three residents who were particularly challenging to the staff. It turned out that once the residents were engaged in activities that were meaningful and pleasurable to them, the behaviors staff had had trouble with abated. Seeing what worked with these residents gave staff ideas about how to brainstorm what might work with other residents. When change is done successfully, it opens the door to new possibilities.

Use "Experiential" Learning

For adults, experience is the best classroom. Covey said that people learn more from what they see modeled than what they hear taught.

St. Camillus wanted to use its van more, but its larger goal was to activate staff's ability to work together for change. Graves and Godfrey taught process improvement to their staff by having the staff take on real situations and work through them together. So the managers talked personally with all the staff to find out what areas the staff felt needed some work. More use of the van was one. Another was making the hallways less of a work area and more of a living space. On each shift, staff took responsibility for figuring out with co-workers ways to make the space more functional for them and the residents. Graves and Godfrey met regularly with the staff about their ideas as they held discussions with their co-workers, designed plans, and implemented them. They learned how to factor in issues they wouldn't have thought of, or remembered if they'd been given in a memo. They learned how to work issues through with co-workers to arrive at solutions that worked for everybody. They learned how to change by working on real change. They were then ready to take on the next challenge.

This is also known as unit-based quality improvement, or *ground-up* problem solving. One home decided to change its quality assurance process from a top-down to a ground-up approach. The old practice had been for the QA committee to review the data, identify areas of concern, and schedule in-service training for staff working where the problems were occurring. They pilot tested a new ground-up approach. On the unit with the highest number of people with pressure ulcers, the nurse pulled staff together to discuss each person who had a pressure ulcer and figure out what could be contributing to the situation. Then they talked about possible interventions. The staff talked from shift to shift about what might work and continued those conversations as they succeeded in healing all the pressure ulcers and preventing any new ones from occurring. They learned through experience what they needed to do and worked together to do it.

They also learned that the further away from the point of care their meeting was, the less likely it was to be successful in addressing the true causes of the problem in a way that would actually work. Not only did the unit-staff learn how to apply quality improvement to their daily resident care, but also the management team learned how to restructure its quality improvement processes to be "ground-up." See Box 6.1 for information about a resource on "ground-up" process improvement.

Create a Climate Where the Truth Can Be Heard

The main ingredient in deep transformative change is an ability to truly hear from people and to include both residents and staff in the process. This kind of leadership puts decisions in the hands of the people most affected by how things are—the residents and those closest to them.

Inclusion is not for the faint of heart. You have to be prepared to hear things that other people see differently from you. By including people, we get to know the downside to any new idea as well as the upside. It is only in knowing the downside that we can proactively address it. And by including people, you get to the solution in a way that everyone feels comfortable going forward with.

People want things to go well. They need to be able to trust the process, and trust that they'll have a voice in it.

Too often staff's legitimate concerns are mislabeled as resistance.

Box 6.1
Ground-Up Performance Improvement

A resource for ground-up performance improvement is *Getting Better All the Time: Working Together for Continuous Improvement: A Guide for Nursing Home Staff* by Isabella and Cobble Hill Nursing Center in New York City. It is available on their websites: www.isabella.org and www.cobblehill.org. It identifies the following elements:

- Unit-based analysis of problems and identification of solutions

- Education to support process improvement skills among frontline staff

- Use of systems for process improvement that are easily accessible to hands-on staff, such as change of shift meetings, rounds, and other unit-based meetings

- Access to and management of data among staff directly involved in and affected by the area for improvement

- Integration of quality of life considerations into quality of care issues

- Interdepartmental and interdisciplinary collaboration

- Ground-up problem-solving approach by clinical leads and nursing leads

What staff are resisting is being ignored when they see real problems that they don't know will be listened to or addressed. If staff voice concerns, take out a flipchart and make a list of all the concerns. Tell the staff that their concerns provide a roadmap of what needs to be addressed to make the change successfully. Then engage staff in thinking through how to address each concern.

In his book *Good to Great*, Jim Collins talks about one of the foundational pieces of moving from good to great being "creating a climate where the truth can be heard." It is true, we really do need to create a space where we include people to the point where they can tell us what is going wrong as well as what is going right.

One administrator, as he was trying to bring frontline workers into conversation, recognized that he had to level the playing field for them if he wanted them to feel fully included. So at the beginning of his meetings, he had a basket in the middle of the table and he asked staff, as they came in, to remove their name badges and put them in the basket before they began the meeting. This act was a symbolic way of making sure everyone felt their contributions had equal value regardless of their position in the organization.

Collins identified four key practices with which to create a climate for true dialogue:

1. Pay attention to red flags.

2. Conduct autopsies without blame.

3. Engage in dialogue and debate, not coercion.

4. Lead with your questions not your answers.

It all starts with a genuine belief that staff have the answers. One of the administrators who successfully guided her nursing home through months of tricky situations after Hurricane Katrina said that it was a team effort that got them through, and that they continued that approach after the crisis abated. She and her DON commented:

> Everyone's opinion counts. We may be the ones that are the leaders, but sometimes they have better ideas than we do. And you realize that I may be a little smarter than you on this, but you are a little bit smarter than me on that. Everyone has something to offer. And you value their opinion. We have carried that forward a lot since we have been back.

As Covey said, a quality process depends on the people side of the process, that the people most affected by the change are involved in shaping, implementing, and evaluating it.

So, the how of change is not just about a process of change. It is also about a way of leading. In everyday practice, draw on staff's insights. When that is the culture of your workplace, you'll be able to draw people into any change process and tap into their wisdom and contributions.

The How of High Involvement

To be effective, efforts should not be designed or implemented by the management team in isolation. A process that involves a wide spectrum of staff is a key ingredient for success. Staff know what is working and what is not. You'll be more on target in what you do and more effective in doing it if representatives of the entire staff are involved along the way.

Being involved in problem solving starts by having regular staff engagement in the day-to-day routine. Start and end your shifts together with a brief stand-up meeting to share information. Build a shift overlap into the schedule so staff personally hand off care of their residents. Use the time to identify problem areas and engage in group problem solving. This is a basic means of fostering teamwork, shared knowledge, and mutual respect. This may seem impossible in your current environment, with people hurrying to finish their work at the end of their shift, and incoming staff racing to answer call lights. However, a smooth hand-off between shifts and a stand-up to start and end the shift are the best way to have good continuity of care, to maintain consistency in attending to residents' needs, and to have good working relationships across shifts. Once staff get in the habit of coming together at the beginning and end of the shift, everyone will willingly join in because they will see the value and come to rely on that time together. The cost of intershift overlap will pay for itself to the point that you will realize you can't afford not to build in that kind of communication.

The large urban home that made dramatic changes in its care practices used its shift overlap time as the place to meet with other disciplines and departments to discuss how to take on the changes. Other clinicians joined in with the staff to talk about areas that needed attention and how they could help. This is the best time for the sharing of timely, accurate, problem-solving–oriented information that is necessary for good working relationships.

Starting and ending the shift together is a good starting point for having staff meet regularly to troubleshoot. It gets staff into a mode of huddling to problem solve. Stephen R. Covey wrote, "Sometimes transformation requires no outside control—when people are given the space to open up, they often unravel their own problems and solutions become clear in the process." Bring staff information so they can look at how to implement evidence-based "best practices." Collect and share performance data with unit-based staff. This includes human resource data, clinical outcomes, and business results. Give staff benchmark information and help them compare their results with those benchmarks. Facilitate real root cause analysis that is person specific. Ask for staff's thoughts on interventions. Ask what they need from the organization to be able to carry those interventions out. Come back regularly with updated information and celebrate their accomplishments.

Use these meetings to look at residents who are declining or could benefit from interventions to support improvements. Look at resident assessment data on an ongoing basis as a guide. Bringing this kind of information and problem-solving orientation into these meetings turns them from routine exchanges of rote information into venues for critical thinking and quality improvement.

Change-of-shift meetings, care-planning meetings, unit-based problem solving—all these build staff's experience with collaborative problem solving so that they can be comfortably involved in organizationwide activities.

Committees

A good way to have high involvement is to activate a committee. For the committee to be successful it must include employees from all strata of the organization who have an interest in and are willing to work to make a difference in this area. It also has to have someone who is a formal decision maker in the home, such as the administrator, DON, or committee leader who has been given decision-making authority by the administration. If the workgroup or committee doesn't have someone with decision-making authority as a member, build in regular meetings with decision makers every step of the way so that the group continually knows they are on the right track.

Committees need to feel that their efforts are meaningful. If their work is later vetoed, they will be hesitant to join in future efforts. Be clear with a committee about what it is charged to do, what permission it has, and what parameters it must abide by.

To make the most of this committee, operate it in a way that gives everyone an opportunity to contribute and everyone an opportunity to learn and grow. When McDonald's staff committee worked on improving the way they supported each other when residents died, all the staff had an opportunity to learn. They divided duties. Some committee members called other homes in the area, others called hospice, some interviewed residents, families, and co-workers. They all learned more about the possibilities and became actively engaged in figuring out what would work best at Glenridge.

Steps for good participation in a committee include the following:

1. Make personal invitations to your frontline and supervisory staff to encourage their participation. Think about a good mix, with representation across departments and shifts.

2.   Communicate facility-wide that you are recruiting for this committee and that all are welcome to participate.

3.   Schedule meetings when members can attend, especially those on evenings and nights. In order to support participation by staff who don't work the day shift, have some committee meetings during other times of day or create mechanisms for staff to communicate with those who work different shifts.

4.   Make sure everyone knows when the meetings are scheduled to happen by personally letting each person and their supervisor know.

5.   Arrange coverage so staff can participate without adding to their own or their co-workers' stress. One option is to have someone from management cover responsibilities on the floor during the meeting. While management staff routinely go to meetings, staff with hands-on responsibilities will be worried about what they didn't get done, left for others, or awaits them when they get back. Or they may not be able to come unless they know their responsibilities are covered.

6.   Make it worth people's time—listen to what they have to say, act on their suggestions, and follow through on what you say you will do.

A Step-by-Step Committee Approach

1.   *Start by having everyone expand their perspectives.* At the nursing home preparing to move from a very old, crowded building into a brand new living space, staff were discussing how to help residents move their belongings. The problem was that not all of their belongings would fit in the new rooms. At first the discussion centered on how to help residents shed their "excess belongings." To get started, the staff did an exercise in which they listed the 10 items they would want to take with them into a nursing home if they needed to move into one. They were told to cross off 3 items, then another 2. They had a very hard time crossing off items. This gave them empathy for what residents were experiencing and led them to discuss the connection between one's belongings and their well-being. Putting themselves in the residents' position changed their focus so that they started to explore ways to help residents keep the possessions that were meaningful to them.

2. *Look at root causes of problems.* Break into small groups to have committee members talk about and list out on a flip chart all of the reasons that they think the problem is happening. People will be more engaged and freer to voice their opinions in a small group conversation than in a large one. Small groups also level the playing field, while in large groups frontline staff tend to defer to formal leaders. This is crucial to the effectiveness of your process. If staff hold back, the group can easily go down a path that doesn't get to the heart of the matter. When staff are free to think critically about what is going on, they can guide the process to address the true causes. Give sufficient time for people to really think this through. As a whole group, talk about the lists that each group has generated. Look both at areas where there seems to be a lot of agreement and at areas that only a few people have mentioned. Committee members will learn more about these areas as they take the discussion to others.

3. *Take the conversation out to the whole organization.* Often committee members think they are supposed to deliberate in a vacuum and have all the answers. Committees work most effectively when they seek information and opinions from their peers. Give each committee member assignments of people to talk with and/or topics to find out more about from these conversations. Talk with residents and staff about their needs and ideas. Inform supervisors and managers that committee members have these assignments and will need time to complete them. Let others on staff know that this is happening, and encourage them to participate in interviews to give their input. Give the committee enough time to complete these assignments before meeting again. Check in with committee members between meetings to make sure they are progressing.

4. *Look at what you've learned and set priorities for action.* At the next meeting ask each person to share what he or she has learned. Take time to sift through the information. This is not a time to take a vote or let some people's viewpoints trump others. It is a time to gather all the aspects of the situation. If a problem is being addressed, take a comprehensive look at the causes of a problem and possible interventions. If the group is assigned to initiate new activity, such as a better welcome for new residents, look at what will be involved in putting any plans in place. Start with easy

wins that can have a positive impact—what is realistic and easy to do that can have an immediate positive result. Some areas may take longer to address. Keep these in mind so that as you take your first actions, you do so in a way that begins to address the larger issues as well.

5.   *Pilot test, adjust, then spread.* Start with small pilot tests of change. Allow for a trial and error process on a small scale. Take committee assignments to check in with people about how it is working. Make adjustments as needed, and when it is working, spread what you've done and build on it.

Putting It All Together: The How of Change

The following are core elements of a successful change process:

1.   *Draw from personal experience:* What do you know from your own experience? Ask yourself, "What would I need if I were in this situation?"

2.   *Look at the current situation:* Try to be objective, and step back to look at what you are you doing now. Find out what people are experiencing. Lie in a resident's bed for 15 minutes with your eyes closed and note the sounds, smells, and feel of the experience. Or stay overnight. Ask staff about their experience and perspective.

3.   *Decide what needs to change:*
     • Keep what is good, what is working. Often staff fear that a change means everything will be tossed. Take a strength-based approach, building on what works well.
     • Look at what is identified as not working. If it is not working for staff or residents, it is probably not working for your organization, though its negative impact may not be obvious. Get more information about why it is not working, so that you know what impact it is having and what about it needs to be fixed. When everyone is aware of the negative impact, it is easier to agree to make a change.
     • For each area that needs to change, figure out whether it is a function that is still needed, and if so, how it can be done in a better way that will support stability. *Sifting through what is working and not working will help you ensure that in the course of change, you don't lose the good or lose sight of the necessary.*

4. *Do it in stages.* As a team, review the list *of areas where change is needed.* Determine what is easy to do and what is more complex. Identify areas that will have a strong positive impact. Figure out which changes can be stepping stones to future changes.

5. *Prioritize to start where you can easily implement something, have the best chance of success, and have a positive impact.* You're building your capacity for change as you're taking on each change, so approach the process developmentally.

6. *Explain to all staff what you're doing and why.* Staff need to understand the reasoning, and know that this is thought out. They need to be able to ask questions and contribute to determining the answers.

7. *Enlist staff participation.* As staff agree to become involved, have them work to bring in the experiences and ideas of their co-workers. Sometimes one or two CNAs are asked to sit on a committee and "represent" their co-workers. Having everyone on the committee actively solicit the perspectives of everyone involved is a better way to have true staff engagement and a true understanding of people's viewpoints.

8. *Collect data to measure your impact.* Ask staff how they would know something is better or worse, and then have them involved in gathering the baseline information and monitoring as they go along. This way they will know for themselves what is working, and they can see red flags right away.

9. *Evaluate each effort and make midcourse adjustments as you go along.* Nothing works perfectly on the first try. And everything can continually improve. Too often people think they are done when they phase out of planning into implementation. However, allowing time afterward to make adjustments is what will ensure your success. Staff often fear that things will go wrong and they'll be stuck with a flawed process. Once they know that you will see it through with them, they'll be more willing to give it a try.

10. *Announce progress and celebrate positive results.* When everyone has the data, everyone can see the results. As midcourse adjustments succeed and improvements become clear, let everyone know your appreciation and celebrate their accomplishments. If you are able

to fix early implementation problems, include that information in the results you share.

11. *Build on the gains you have achieved.* Take on the next area. As you go forward, *maintain your previous efforts,* or you may soon experience a backward slide. You'll start to build momentum in a positive direction. As staff feels the immediate benefits of the changes, they'll be more eager and receptive for your next effort.

12. *Use a "high involvement" approach:*

    • Involve staff in identifying what is going on and identifying solutions, implementing solutions, and evaluating whether they're working.
    • Some staff will be better at this than others. Make this an educational experience in which employees learn how to use their problem-solving skills for organizational improvement.

There is a 2000-year-old Chinese poem that serves as a good guide to this high-involvement approach:

> Go to the people
> Learn from them
> Love them
> Start with what they know
> Build on what they have
> But the best of leaders
> When their task is accomplished
> When their work is done
> The people will remark:
> "We have done it ourselves."
> —Lao Tzu, *The Book of the Way,* 600 BC–531 BC

## CHAPTER 7

Moving the Flywheel— Getting Traction

DURING THE YEAR DOCUMENTED by his journal, David Farrell counted 133 changes, small and large, that all contributed to the organization's success. From getting indoor plants, painting the graffiti, fixing broken chairs, getting softer toilet paper, and switching to bendable straws, to replacing his director of nursing (DON), holding regular community meetings, establishing a mentor program, and moving Mr. Waitts, each of Farrell's changes contributed momentum to take on further changes and achieve continually better results.

Now a regional director of operations, Farrell brings leaders of the homes he works with together to conduct a root cause analysis of their successes. Accomplishments aren't magical. They are the result of applying specific practices. He helps his administrators and directors of nursing look at why they succeeded, so they can succeed again. This is called *meta-cognition*—it means *knowing what you know*. When changes work, take the time to figure out why, so that you can do it again. Make sure to maintain your successes; it is easy to slide back into former patterns and then slide back into former results. It is also easy to maintain momentum. Successes open up new possibilities. When you take the time to look at what you're doing and why it is working, you gain insights that help you build on your successes and tackle the next logical area. As staff see the possibilities, they eagerly join in to take on positive changes.

This chapter provides some starting points that will give you traction in moving the flywheel forward. As you move the flywheel it will generate momentum for further changes. Start with staff stability, reducing stress, and building a positive chain of leadership. These interventions give you the foundation for taking on more complex changes to individualize care, improve your clinical outcomes, and increase resident, family, and staff satisfaction. As you improve your clinical care and satisfaction, your census will improve. As your census improves you will have more resources that you can pump back into your building to make further improvements.

Figure 7.1 is our roadmap for successful change. In this road map, focus on people first, and then on systems that support people to work well together. Let people know the importance of good working relationships by modeling genuine caring. Voice your expectation that staff use good interpersonal skills, and compliment people for their caring ways. Hire people with good interpersonal skills. Put systems in place, such as start-of-shift stand-up meetings, to nurture and support good working relationships. The first two parts of our book provide guidance for creating a positive chain of leadership and achieving staff stability. In this chapter, we focus on areas that help you build on the foundation of staff stability to achieve high performance as an organization. We discuss ways to strengthen systems that support people to work well together, reduce stress so staff energy can be used positively, and individualize care practices to improve outcomes and satisfaction.

Throughout this chapter, we rely on the theory of relational coordination as a guide in our work. Relationships are the foundation

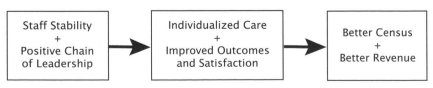

Figure 7.1.
Roadmap for Successful Change.

for good care, for good teamwork, and for effective organizations. Organizations thrive when their systems support good teamwork. To strengthen your organization's relational coordination, reinvigorate key processes you already have in place including start-of-shift and shift hand-off processes, interdisciplinary care planning, and quality improvement efforts.

Relational Coordination

The theory suggests that relationships with the resident are shaped by the relationships among all those who are caring for the resident. It is the *community* of relationships that shapes the resident's experience. Echoing Stephen Covey's people paradigm, relational coordination finds that outcomes for residents are shaped by the effectiveness of coordination and communication among staff. This communication depends on the quality of the underlying relationships.

The quality of relationships and communication is particularly important in settings like nursing homes, with high levels of task interdependence, uncertainty, and time constraints. For example, relationships between CNAs, nurses, and food service staff can affect how easily a resident can have an alternate meal or mealtime. In nursing homes, almost every aspect of care is affected by the actions of people from different departments. Being able to make occasional or systematic changes depends on the ability of staff across departments and functions to work well together, with a shared understanding of why a change is needed by residents.

The effectiveness of an organization's systems and practices in supporting relational coordination is measured by the factors related to its communication and relationships. Is communication frequent, timely, accurate, and oriented to problem solving? Do relationships reflect shared goals, shared knowledge, mutual respect, and a sense of a common purpose? Look at what mechanisms are in place to support frequent, problem-solving–oriented communication and relationships. One evening nurse supervisor described her practice of personally checking in with the evening cook every afternoon to make sure they had the same information about any residents newly admitted, returned from the hospital, or no longer there. She said that she had tried emailing, leaving voice messages, and completing the food slips, but that nothing worked as well as talking in person. Now, if she doesn't get down to see the cook, the cook comes and finds her, because they have come to depend on this regular check-in as the most effective way to make sure they have the information they need to provide for their residents.

Effective relational coordination has been associated with enhanced resident quality of life and higher nursing assistant job satisfaction (Jody Hoffer Gittell, *High Performance Healthcare: Using the Power of Relationships to Achieve Quality, Efficiency and Resilience*, 2009). Gittell documented that homes had better resident and staff satisfaction when their staff had the ability and will to relate positively to other people. This included the ability to see the perspective of others, empathize with their situation, and respect the work they do, even if it is of lower status. In successful nursing homes in her study, staff had the ability to see how each individual's work connects to others around the wants and needs of the residents. In general, relationships were valued in the low-turnover homes. This was noticeably absent in the high-turnover facilities.

Good relationships start with people who have good interpersonal skills. People in supervisory roles with good interpersonal skills help their care teams thrive. Mary Lescoe-Long and Michael Long found that the interpersonal skills of supervisors are one of the biggest factors in stability and satisfaction in nursing homes (1998). To foster relational coordination and relational competency, support your supervisors and managers in the development of their people skills. Foster good relationships by hiring people who have good interpersonal skills (see Chapter 2). When staff members don't have those good skills, look to develop their interpersonal abilities through direct discussion, mentoring, and opportunities to grow and learn. Homes participating in a 2010–2011 Critical Access Nursing Home Project sponsored by Advancing Excellence in America's Nursing Homes, found that when they talked with a few of their supervisors who were perceived as negative by their staff, the nurses were at first taken aback, and then responded well by being more conscientious about how they interacted.

Put in place systems such as nurse supervisory meetings to create an environment that supports good interpersonal relationships. One Critical Access Nursing Home decided to institute regular meetings with nurses to talk over their supervisory challenges and give them an opportunity to grow in their abilities by learning from their peers.

Be alert to systems that foster conflict. For example, often conflicts occur between shifts over work not accomplished. When staff rush in or out at shift change, they don't have the opportunity to make a smooth hand-off, and on-coming staff can be resentful of the work left to them by those going off shift. Having staff make rounds together during a change of shift overlap can mitigate the conflict by having staff understand what happened for each resident during the preceding hours. Making rounds together fosters positive relationships across shifts, providing the basis for continuity in resident care and regular problem solving together.

By putting systems in place to foster good working relationships and hiring people with good interpersonal skills, conflicts will decrease and people will work better together. When new employees join a staff of people who work well together, there is more likelihood they'll have a good experience and stay. Reducing stress and putting systems in place that bring out the staff's good interpersonal skills helps staff perform at their best. Then, what may have seemed like a conflict-filled environment changes into one where people work well together. If you then identify a lone individual or two who stand out as continually negative, it will be easier to take action. In fact, the staff will need you to take action with the few people who don't respond to these positive efforts. Jim Collins says one of the worst things you can do to your good employees is to inflict negative co-workers on them.

Use the theory of relational coordination to focus on creating and supporting systems that enable staff to communicate regularly and solve problems together. Key mechanisms for this include change-of-shift report, interdisciplinary care planning, and unit-based quality improvement efforts. When these systems work well, everyone performs at their best.

Change of Shift

Overlap shifts so that staff coming on and going off can talk directly about each resident in their care. While this may seem expensive, the lack of overlap creates costly errors. Expand change-of-shift report from an exchange of limited medical information to a full discussion of each resident's experiences that day. Focus as much on quality-of-life factors as on quality-of-care factors. Use the resident assessment tool, MDS 3.0 (Minimum Data Set), as a guide to check in on each resident's mood, cognition, and functional ability. Hone in on ways to prevent risks and promote improvements. Take extra time discussing any residents who are new so that staff can share with co-workers about the resident's background, personality, daily routines, and ways to support their sense of well-being.

Look for ways to foster interdisciplinary and interdepartmental collaboration. Have consistently assigned staff from housekeeping and food service regularly participate in change-of-shift stand-up meetings so that everyone shares information about how residents are doing. Have the director of maintenance join each unit's meeting periodically to hear about and be able to troubleshoot any issues that are causing stress and can be resolved. For example, is the timing for garbage pickup leaving units with overflowing cans after dinner? Would it help to replenish the linen on a different schedule? Is staff using a particular piece of equipment in a manner that is causing it to break frequently?

Change of shift is the venue for regular, timely information sharing and creative thinking. It is also a forum for interdisciplinary care planning and "ground-up" quality improvement.

Interdisciplinary Assessment and Care Planning

If your assessment and care planning process is more a burden than a tool, you are not alone. The typical process can feel far removed from the realities of day-to-day care, with little impact on it or input from those living closest to it. The meetings themselves often become rote paperwork exercises. The resident assessment coordinator is left to review CNA and charge nurse notes that often contain unexplained inconsistencies, in an effort to complete what feels like an onerous form, the Minimum Data Set (MDS) 3.0. Errors can be costly in terms of financial reimbursement, though the cost to residents and staff of having such a burdensome and irrelevant process is even higher. This type of assessment and care planning process provides an excellent example of the burdens when relational coordination is lacking.

MDS 3.0 works best when used by the staff most directly involved in the daily care and support of each resident. If you align CNA flow sheets with MDS 3.0 documentation, and have consistently assigned staff who know each resident well, CNAs can note and document daily any changes in resident's mood, functional status, or other developments. For example, CNAs can note if there is even a subtle change in bed mobility, appetite, or ways of relating to others. When staff see the connection between their documentation and residents' well-being, the documentation becomes meaningful because staff know what they are looking for and why.

Build relational coordination into your assessment and care planning process by using MDS-aligned flow sheets to review each resident in CNA-to-CNA change of shift hand-off and identify any variations from the norm. For example, when were the change in resident's bed mobility, appetite, and relations first noted, and how long have they been going on?

In noting any changes, CNAs and charge nurses can identify action needed to mitigate potential risks and support potential improvements, and plan for the day's care. For example, staff could discuss what could be causing the change in mobility and what to do about it. If the resident is more independent, ask how this improvement can be supported. If the resident is less independent, is it because of weakness from lack of appetite? Do all these changes add up to a greater concern? What are the risks?

This paves the way for unit-based, interdisciplinary problem solving. CNAs and charge nurses can coordinate daily resident needs with other disciplines and departments to implement individualized care interventions. For example, is a change needed in the timing of physical therapy or of meals or in the type of food for the resident?

These are times to find individualized approaches and catch iatrogenic practices (declines caused by the organization's approach rather than by the natural progression of a resident's condition). At one nursing home where a man often struck out at other residents, staff learned from his social history that he had been used to a very physically engaged life working outdoors. They realized that he never got outside and never had any constructive physical outlets. Once they understood what he needed, they were able to devise an approach that gave him positive ways to use his energy and reduced his violent outbursts. Prior to having the discussion with the unit staff, the interdisciplinary care planning team had ineffectively repeated care plan goals stating that the resident would not have violent outbursts. By having the discussion on the unit, with the regular caregiving staff, the team was able to relieve the man's distress, and the distress of other residents affected by his previous violence. Residents' outcomes will improve when they can pursue what feels normal to them, and follow their own schedules and daily habits.

So often, residents' declines are accelerated by the institutional environment. Use daily care planning on the unit, and inclusive care planning meetings to actively reexamine care plan goals. Are they your goals or the resident's goals? In the case of the man who'd always had outdoor physical work, his goal, as developed by the care team, had been to stop hitting others. By framing the care goal as something he needed to *stop* doing rather than something they needed to *start* doing to help him get what he needed, the care goals had failed to be met, quarter after quarter. Only by understanding his needs and meeting them were they able to recognize his outbursts as calls for help, and respond immediately with useful interventions.

The common practice now of rote reviews in which goals are repeated despite their lack of success makes the whole process a drain on time without a positive impact. When a resident exhibits distressing behaviors, the goal should be to find out what is causing the resident distress and what can alleviate it. Old "behavior modification" approaches are rarely successful and yet they are too often carried forward from one care plan to the next, even as they continue to be unmet. Have true dialogue among clinicians with residents, their families, and their consistent caregiver to problem solve together. Seek to understand what anxiety or need has been triggered and how to meet it. If goals are unmet, time and again, are they the right goals?

Homes that integrate resident assessment and care planning into daily practice get more accurate information about a resident's condition and about successful approaches to care. As staff know residents well through consistent assignment, they tune in to subtle resident changes.

CNAs are more likely to chart accurately when the information is useful and there are regular forums for using it. Aligning CNA flow sheets with elements of MDS 3.0 so that staff routinely use the scales in MDS 3.0 to document changes, prompts staff to notice and make note of them. CNAs are then familiar with the medical terminology being used to categorize residents' conditions and are able to be specific in their documentation to provide the information necessary to code accurately. This creates alignment between charting and coding and saves all the time now currently spent correcting one or the other.

Capturing variations, risks, and potential through discussions at start and end of shift, and in shift change hand-off, helps staff focus in on any variations and be alert regarding any risks or potential improvements. When staff catch situations early and can figure out how to tailor interventions to each person, they more likely can prevent or turn around a bad situation, or successfully support progress. Making the assessment and care planning process a part of daily care leads to better care outcomes because staff are able to address situations quickly, consistently, and effectively across shifts. Residents improve more rapidly and have slower and less decline and fewer negative events.

Good outcomes mean good surveys. By providing individualized attention to residents' needs, preferences, changes, risks, and potential, homes will be better positioned to meet the federal standard "to attain or maintain the highest practicable physical, mental, and psychosocial well-being of each resident." (OBRA '87 [Omnibus Budget Reconciliation Act of 1987]). When staff provide accurate comprehensive documentation of the work they do on forms that are aligned with MDS 3.0 codes, their work will be recognized and paid for. For example, if staff on some shifts are giving residents extensive assistance getting in or out of bed, or providing cuing or other interventions due to residents' cognitive losses, they will only be paid for this work if they write it down.

Tying assessment and care planning into daily work and life invigorates care-planning meetings with reality and relevance. If staff are actively engaged in thinking critically about each resident's progress, they will be more able to contribute to the care planning process. Set up your systems to make this contribution a reality. Have your care plan meeting on the unit where the resident lives, at a time and place convenient to the resident, family, and certified nursing assistant (CNA). Make your care plan meeting environment and format comfortable and inviting. Too often, it feels to CNAs, residents, and families more like a trip to the principal's office than a forum for real open exchange and exploration. When the care plan process is a natural extension of daily discussion on the floor, CNAs are more easily able to contribute.

Instead of thinking of care planning as a quarterly event, see it as a part of everyday conversation among staff who routinely huddle together to discuss how residents are doing and what they need. The assessment process was never meant to be done in a corner office by a staff member with access to a computer who inputs often contradictory notes from nurses and from CNA flow sheets. The intent was to have an ongoing process of discussion among people closest to a resident, for facilitating positive care and life for each resident. The further apart your assessment and care planning process is from the daily life of the resident and those providing resident care, the less relevant it is. Who can afford to fill out complex paperwork in a way that is not relevant to daily care? Or to track staff down for explanations of inconsistencies in their charting? When your MDS process is integrated into the daily fabric of staff work on the unit, the information will be accurate. This "ground-up" approach also increases the likelihood that your MDS data and your caregivers' charting will be aligned, that staff will understand the importance of what they are documenting because they will actively use the information to note changes, risks, and opportunities for the residents they care for. This alignment means that your MDS process will also more likely capture the work in a way that generates the care residents need and brings you the payment you are entitled to.

Quality Improvement

Most organizations operate their quality improvement (QI) efforts at the organizational level with a strictly clinical focus. To get real traction for your quality improvement activity, focus on each individual resident and bring the QI process to the staff where the resident lives. The further away from the resident and caregiving staff a QI effort is, the less relevance, accuracy, or possibility of success you will have. While it is important to have an organization-wide understanding of trends and performance, it is only by zeroing in on each person, with the staff who care for that person, that you will be able to put in place an effective approach.

Broaden your focus to include quality of life factors in considering your clinical protocols. If you are worried about a resident at risk for pressure ulcers who isn't eating well, find out why she isn't eating and make adjustments in how food is available. Does the person want smaller meals more often, different food, a quieter or more engaged environment for eating, times of day that are more in line with lifelong routines? Pay attention to residents' individual routines in designing interventions. Food supplements don't address the root cause of why a person isn't eating; they merely make up for the loss of nutrients. Identify individual indicators of how a resident is doing.

Use a ground-up approach, with unit-based staff doing the problem solving. Staff know residents intimately. They know their patterns, their moods, their needs. If residents are developing pressure ulcers, don't have your first intervention be to send staff to a class on pressure ulcer prevention. Meet with them right where they work, and look together at all the factors that could be contributing to the skin breakdown. Elicit their ideas for interventions. Understand the barriers they face in implementing these interventions. Facilitate the sharing of strategies across shifts for a full 24/7 perspective and to ensure continuity of effort.

Often interventions need cooperation from other departments. Involve representatives from each area affected by a problem or a potential solution. If a resident needs meals on a different schedule, food service and housekeeping staff will have to work with CNAs and nursing to implement a new schedule. With this approach staff can identify root causes and effective interventions.

For unit-based, ground-up problem solving, focus first on every unit's shift hand-off because this is where staff share the most timely and individualized information about each resident and about the care area as a whole. Inject critical thinking and collaborative problem solving into this process. Critical thinking is fostered by consistent assignment, through which staff get to know residents so well that they can immediately spot subtle changes that warrant further examination. Critical thinking is also fostered by regular huddles, start-of-shift stand-up and shift change meetings where staff thoughtfully review how each resident is doing. These systems create an environment in which critical thinking can flourish.

Use unit-based process improvement to kick-start your change process. If you'd like to improve how residents experience the first 24 to 72 hours so that they get off to a good start in their stay with you, talk it through first on the units. Invite staff from other departments to join in the discussion. Identify common areas of concern that can be addressed, such as making sure the food service staff learn about a resident's arrival so no meals are missed. Work out a system for notifying the kitchen, even when residents arrive long after they were expected, so that they do not have to wait for food. If you want to decentralize food service so that many foods are available right in residents' living area, talk through with unit-based staff, housekeepers, and dietary staff just how it will work. Use change-of-shift meetings to check in and make adjustments as needed.

Change-of-shift meetings, an interdisciplinary assessment and care-planning process, unit-based problem solving—all build staff's experience with collaborative problem solving so that they can be comfortably involved in organizationwide activities. These organizational practices foster relational coordination because they provide mechanisms for frequent, timely, problem-solving–oriented communication based on shared goals, shared knowledge, and mutual respect.

Reduce Stress

Sustained stress has significant negative consequences. While we were working with homes recovering from Hurricane Katrina, we were joined for one educational session by a local organization providing counseling and other supports. The organization's representative held up a packet of Sweet and Lo and said it was the object of a physical altercation in the employee break room at one nursing home he had visited. He explained that on a stress scale of 1 to 10, once people are higher than 7, their tolerance is worn thin. If they are at 9 or 10 for a sustained period of time, their tolerance is eroded even further. In this nursing home something as simple as the last Sweet and Lo was beyond what the employees could tolerate. Since then, as we've worked with nursing homes throughout the country, we've asked people regularly what their stress level is. We frequently hear people rate themselves between 7 and 10, and sometimes even off the charts.

We now know from brain studies that long-term stress erodes executive function and memory. Long-term stress makes complex reasoning harder. Tolerance, patience, and flexibility become brittle.

Staff work hard enough. If there are stresses that are within your control to relieve, make that your priority. When staff are relieved of some stresses, they can work better together and figure out how to make things better. Farrell did a root cause analysis at one home to understand why two staff members had come to blows with each other. They were fighting over use of the one working sit-to-stand machine. He told the management team, *we caused the fight, because we didn't have enough equipment for the staff when they needed it.* Farrell's mantra is "anything to reduce stress." Make sure you have enough equipment and supplies. Look at workflow to find ways to help staff save steps.

At a home designated by the state survey agency as a Special Focus Facility because of its long history of serious problems, the new administrator focused immediately on building trust with employees, stabilizing staffing, and reducing stress. She got staff the supplies they needed to do their jobs, and with her management team was out on the floor pitching in. She acknowledged people's contributions with lots of sincere and frequent appreciation, even sending staff cards to express her thanks. She identified the need for new positions and made some staffing changes. Even the new maintenance director contributed to creating a more supportive environment. He checked the ventilation system and saw that between the dirty filters and poorly functioning equipment, 90% of the airflow was blocked. Getting clean air was an invisible, yet noticeable, stress reducer.

To anchor staff stability, the administrator brought all levels of staff into key committees focused on improving care and life in the organization. At first, staff members were hesitant, but they soon became more involved. They all took pride in the better results they had on their next few surveys, because they had all contributed to the improvements. This contributed to a higher census. With census up and deficiencies down, staffing stable and good systems firmly in place, the home's turnaround is well on its way.

Nursing homes are fragile ecosystems and, as such, are highly susceptible to subtle changes. And each change affects not only the area being changed, but has a ripple effect throughout the home. When you make a positive change, you are in effect creating an upward spiral. When people work better together they have the energy to take on other changes. Mornings are a good example. When staff have a better start to their day and help when they feel overwhelmed, it carries over into the whole day and into the evening as well.

One way to get a better start to the day is to rethink the use of suppositories. They are overused in many nursing homes and make for a miserable start to the day for residents, CNAs, nurses, housekeepers, and laundry staff. They add an unnecessary layer of stress at an already busy time. Their overuse also compromises residents' ability to remain continent of bowel.

We know that the best ways to address constipation are fiber, fluid, and exercise. We also know what contributes to constipation. Many medications that reduce anxiety or encourage sleep also make bowels sluggish. Inactivity, lack of appetite, and low fluid intake make it worse. When suppositories are used, residents awaken to a deeply unpleasant experience, which is also unpleasant for the CNAs tending to them and the nurses administering them. Sustained use of suppositories causes people to lose their muscle function and their ability to eliminate independently. This, like many other practices, reflects the norm in the field, and so it is hard to see how to do something different.

One nursing home that was looking to change to "gentle awakening," where residents would get up in the morning on their own instead of being awakened for morning care, recognized that it could reduce its use of suppositories and improve mornings for everyone. They focused on suppositories after reviewing an incident report about a resident who hit his caregiver when he was awakened at 4:00 a.m. to have a suppository administered. They did a root cause analysis and realized that suppositories were routinely given as a protocol. As they talked through the problem, they realized that they could explore avenues that were more natural and in tune with human needs. With good teamwork, they were able to increase fiber, fluid, and exercise for many of their residents by individualizing their care and meal routines. They reduced their suppository use by a third. The reduction in suppositories also reduced stress and freed up staff to be more flexible in meeting their residents' individualized needs in the morning because one contributor to the hectic pace of the morning had been eliminated.

Such changes not only benefit residents, they also relieve stress for staff and contribute to staff stability. Many stressors can be reduced by taking a look at a situation with an open mind rather than being stuck with "how it's always been done." Through a common-sense, ground-up approach, the people who provide the care can easily figure out better solutions—to everyone's benefit. As many homes explore ways to decentralize and "de-schedule" food service, they find that by talking it through with staff, they can ease the rush hour experience of having to get everyone up at once to be in time for a narrow window of breakfast service. With the same staff using their time differently, the same amount of work gets done, with more benefit to residents and less stress for everyone. This is an enormous benefit. And as stress is relieved, it is easier to take on new challenges.

Implement All Hands on Deck

"All hands on deck" is a management strategy whereby managers help out hands-on caregiving staff during the busiest times of day. While this is not a long-term substitute for having enough staff, helping out during high-stress, labor intensive, times has a number of benefits:

- Residents' care needs are better met.

- Staff stress is relieved.

- Managers get firsthand knowledge of the workload and workplace dynamics.

- Managers role-model teamwork.

- The practice builds different and better relationships with staff.

- It breaks the cycle of staff instability.

It can be beneficial in homes with high turnover or absenteeism, where staff are stressed, as they try to meet residents' needs when they are not fully staffed. Even when homes have a full complement of staff, they may find times during the day that are extremely labor intensive and stressful. When managers pitch in during these high-stress and labor-intensive times, they signal that they care about staff and residents, and they provide tangible help that makes the day go better for residents and staff.

This is an extreme intervention and not a substitute for additional staffing. It is important not to mask the problem of understaffing but instead to use this approach as a bridge to better staffing. It serves as a bridge by reducing the unscheduled absences that come from staff stress, building teamwork so that staff work better together, and providing the management with a firsthand feel for how the work flows and where more staff is needed.

In homes with a high degree of stress and instability, implementing "all hands on deck" can be beneficial. Another special-focus facility had a 77% occupancy and 18 of its residents had pressure ulcers. The administrator and DON were each the fourth person to hold their position in as many years. To break the cycle of instability in their building, they made it a part of their daily work to be out of their offices, making rounds throughout the building, pitching in, getting to know people, and identifying what the needs were.

They got the results of a family satisfaction survey in which they were rated discouragingly low in their ability to meet their residents' needs. Because they were always out and about, they knew that their staff was working very hard. The bright spot in the survey was that families felt staff were kind and caring, so the leadership team knew their staff were doing a good job once they could get to people. Instead of ignoring the devastating survey, which would have been easy to do, because they were working very hard, they saw the families' relationship with the staff as an area of strength to build on. They initiated an all-hands-on-deck approach with everyone on the management team pitching in at times when staff said they were needed, helping out as directed. It made an immediate difference. As they stabilized, they focused on developing their nurses' leadership skills and hiring warm, friendly staff. Each improvement gave them momentum for the next.

Under the three previous administrators and DONs, the staff had felt they were on their own, with no support from upper management. They carried the stress of their hectic pace without relief or support. When the management team pitched in, staff felt immediate relief. As they came to know the leadership team was there to support them, they worked better together. Changes to support stability led to improved care. Over the course of 9 months, they stabilized staffing, eliminated all but one pressure ulcer, and improved to 98% occupancy. They went "from a nursing home in need to a nursing home in the lead," as their administrator said in thanking her team for their success.

The first steps the administrator took were relationship-building rounds and all hands on deck. As described in Chapter 1, making regular rounds keeps your finger on the pulse of relationships and workflow in your building. All hands on deck is an intervention to break a vicious cycle of instability and start the flywheel moving in a positive direction. It can also be a way to support staff while initiating an intervention. At the Massachusetts home that decided to eliminate alarms, the management team used all hands on deck to provide extra help to unit-based staff to monitor potential fall hazards and prevent them. The DON taught the management team what to look for and how to respond. Management's presence gave staff the support they needed to change their practices. Within a few weeks they were able to eliminate alarms in the unit with the most falls, and they dramatically reduced falls. While this intervention was originally thought to be a short-term intervention "until the staff felt comfortable," the managers who took up the rounds said it changed they way they walked through the building. They are now always on alert for ways of stepping in to help.

All hands on deck will enable you to stabilize your staffing and develop the leadership skills for a positive chain of leadership among your management team and your supervisors. As you stabilize, you will find that continuing to pitch in regularly continues the atmosphere of teamwork and collaboration. See Box 7.1 for information on how to implement all hands on deck successfully.

Consistent Assignments for Stable Relationships

Another practice that is key to stability and to successful change is consistent assignments of staff. Consistency in relationships and in care starts with consistent assignments. There is ample evidence now that consistent assignments improve clinical, workforce, and organizational outcomes. Consistent assignment means consistently assigning the same caregivers to the same nursing home residents every day, as an ongoing assignment. Rotating assignment means rotating caregivers from one group of residents to the next after a period of time.

Numerous research studies prove that consistent assignment leads

Box 7.1
All Hands on Deck:
Steps for Successful Implementation

- *This is a management intervention.* Managers go first. As staff see management roll up their sleeves and help out during these stressful times, others will follow their lead. However, if managers merely direct non-nursing staff to help rather than committing to provide personal assistance, the directive will generate resentment rather than good will. This is a way of building better relationships, having your finger on the pulse of workflow, and role-modeling teamwork.

- *Find out from staff when and what help is needed.* Meet with staff on each unit and shift to ask when they need what type of assistance. Usually mealtimes are high-stress times. Other labor-intensive times may be the time around shift change when extra help is needed so that the outgoing staff can give reports to the incoming staff. Or help may be needed for transportation to an event in the home or an appointment.

- *Schedule from the top.* Have someone on the management team develop the schedule and communicate it to all units and all management team members.

- *Be reliable and consistent. Set a schedule and keep to it.* Once a promise is made to help, it is essential to keep the promise. Treat time scheduled for helping on the unit as protected time that cannot be interfered with. Make sure to get a substitute from the management team if you are not able to meet your obligation.

- *Report in to the charge nurse to be assigned duties during your assigned time to help.* While you may have agreed-upon tasks, when you come on the unit, you need to find out what is actually needed right then and there. Checking in with the charge nurse ensures that you can be immediately helpful. It also respects the dynamics on the unit and shores up the chain of leadership.

- *Help seven days a week.* Weekend staff need the help as well. While it is harder to arrange to help on weekends, doing so will have an enormous positive impact.

Box 7.1 *continued*

- *Monitor at management team meetings.* At daily stand-up, check in on what managers are doing and finding. While all hands on deck is a way of pitching in, it is also a management strategy that gives managers a finger on the pulse of caregiving and workplace dynamics. Identify strong performers, solid leaders, and people who need more guidance and development. Talk through ways to use the time on the unit to bring out the best in staff. Note areas of stress and brainstorm interventions that can improve workflow, or areas to target for hiring more staff as you are able.

What Types of Assistance to Provide

- *Help at meals.* Many residents need a lot of assistance and eat at a slow pace. Others need to be cued and talked to so that their meal is enjoyable and digestible. There are many meal-related tasks that managers can do to free up CNAs to provide this intensive assistance. Pass trays. Open milk cartons. Pour drinks. Transport people to the dining room. Get substitute meals from the kitchen. Be a companion to a resident who is eating. Answer call bells while staff assist with meals.

- *Answer call bells.* The majority of call bells involve requests for non-nursing assistance. However, should you need to ask for a CNA's help, offer to pick up something that she was doing or ask how you can be of assistance to her.

- *Make fall prevention, comfort rounds, and other check-ins.* Go room to room and ask residents if there is anything they need assistance with. Make sure water pitchers, TV remotes, call bells, and other items are within residents' reach. Do they need a straw, or their water pitcher refilled, or a snack? Does a resident want their face washed at the end of a meal? Untrained staff need to be very careful about ensuring water pitchers are full, straws available, and snacks given. Residents can be diabetic, or unable to have water and a straw due to swallowing problems. Managers need to take their guidance from nursing staff to provide a helping hand.

- *Be a "runner."* Ask unit staff how you can save them some steps. Offer to make the trip to the kitchen for any food substitutes or refills needed. Does the linen need to be restocked?

Box 7.1 *continued*

Who Does It?

- Include all department heads and anyone else who regularly attends your management meetings, such as members of nursing management, heads of the business office, admissions, food services, housekeeping, maintenance, activities, and rehabilitation services.

How Long Is the Time Period for Assistance?

- Carve out increments of 15 to 30 minutes, and make a schedule so that all managers know where they are needed when. You may need some people to help out twice a day in order to have enough people spread out over the busy times on all shifts and all units.

to enhanced relationships; improved staff attendance; improved staff, resident, and family satisfaction; lower staff turnover; improved accuracy and timeliness of screening and assessments; improved clinical outcomes; and improved quality of life. Consistent assignment is what allows for individualized care and good teamwork, because staff know residents so well that they can anticipate their needs and preferences and get into a good, regular rhythm in their own work. Stable assignments are a cornerstone for teamwork. As you put together consistent assignments, you are also putting together the team that will work together. This creates cohesive teams because consistency allows staff to get into a regular rhythm with their co-workers.

Consistent assignments allow staff to get to know the residents very well. They become the experts on a group of residents, and everyone knows that they can go to them for answers. This is empowering and boosts people's self-esteem. In addition, consistent assignments allow for staff to notice the clinical changes early, before it is too late, and to know what interventions have the best chance of working for that person. This is essential to prevent problems and treat them early when they occur, reducing exposure and risk. Also, consistent assignments reduce turnover because they allow staff to form close relationships with the residents. One CNA said, "I think twice about calling out now, because I know that my residents will miss me." Consistency also means that the staff is better able to provide more resident-centered care and enables them to follow the individual routines of their residents, thereby enhancing residents' quality of life (see Box 7.2).

Box 7.2
Research on the Benefits of Consistent Assignment

Some of the existing literature on consistent staff assignment in nursing homes reveals the following:

- C. L. Cox conducted a before-and-after study and found that residents experienced more control and choice and less agitation, while staff reported an improved ability to provide high-quality care.

- M. A. Patchner found that residents had better clinical outcomes and staff provided better care and more awareness of residents' needs. This contributed to lower turnover and lower absenteeism.

- S. Campbell found that residents experienced a reduction in pressure ulcers and increases in functional ability. Staff felt more accountable, and turnover dropped by 29%.

- B. D. Goldman found that staff, residents, and families prefer consistent assignments. Families reported a greater sense of comfort, and staff reported higher satisfaction.

- Mary Lescoe-Long and Michael Long reported on the Family Member Perspective, that they valued staff's personal empathy, "knowing my mom as a person." They said that this knowing only comes about with consistency. Consistent assignments facilitate their getting to know and trust caregivers. It helps them to know who to go to with questions and gives family members peace of mind.

Meanwhile, the evidence against rotating assignments comes from the high rate of burnout among the 80% of homes that still rotate staff. Karl Pillemer found that 70% of CNAs feel burned out some of the time, 60% feel they sometimes treat the residents impersonally, and 40% feel that they have become hardened emotionally.

The success of consistent assignment depends on the process you use to implement it and how well your supervisors facilitate teamwork and problem solving among staff. Assignments have to be fair. They have to be a good match for residents and for staff. Usually the rub on consistent assignment comes when staff members don't want to be "stuck" with a resident who is hard to care for. But quite often one staff member will have a knack with a resident who pushes another staff member's buttons. Staff needs to be able to talk through issues and strategies for residents they find challenging to care for, and have match-ups that play to their strengths.

Use start-of-shift meetings and impromptu huddles to talk through what is going on and get help in meeting residents' needs. Often residents become challenging to care for when the nursing home's systems don't meet their needs. When staff has no flexibility to adjust to residents' needs, they are faced with the behaviors that signal it is not working for the resident without options for how to respond.

Think about the needle on the old phonographs. The scratchy sound when the needle touches the record is akin to the residents' behavioral protest. Yet the needle is merely the end point of the arm, just as the CNAs need to wake up a resident who wants to sleep in is the end point of a system that sends breakfast trays up from the kitchen on a tight schedule with few decent options for food later in the morning. The protest lands on the CNA, who bears the brunt of systems that don't work. Make sure that CNAs are receiving help from other departments through unit-based quality improvement meetings and care-planning meetings so that systems can be adjusted to support individualized care.

When CNAs are consistently assigned to the same residents and learn their routines, they need the operational systems to be flexible to support them in honoring those routines. This starts by having CNAs figure out what they need and talking through how to operationalize new delivery systems. These discussions need to be interdisciplinary—involving food service, housekeeping, activities, and others whose schedules affect the resident's options for the day. Until systems are individualized, staff will be put in a difficult position by consistent assignments, in that they will also know about each resident's needs but not be able to stretch and flex the system to meet the needs. Really paying attention to building in the systemic flexibility to meet residents' needs will alleviate this.

Iatrogenesis—We Caused It

While some changes are driven by government mandates, other changes steadily evolve as practitioners learn new and better ways to provide care and manage their organizations. Anyone who has been in the field for any length of time has seen changes as practice evolves with new knowledge. A simple example is reality orientation. It used to be the standard of practice in nursing home care. It was thought to be the best practice to say to a woman with dementia who wants to go home to make dinner for her husband, "Your husband is dead, so you don't have to make dinner for him." While this was the standard of practice at the time, it had unintended negative consequences as the information came as news to the resident every time, bringing a new shock and grief. There is a medical term for this—*iatrogenic*—which means, *we caused it*. It is the term for situations where actions with the intention to help have negative consequences. In the case of reality orientation, telling a woman with dementia that her husband is dead caused grief and distress that could have been avoided. As practitioners learned that it is better to say, "Tell me about your husband" or "What do you like to fix?" or "Let's see what's for dinner," they updated the standard of practice.

Practice standards in health care continually evolve as we learn better ways of providing care. Some of today's norms will be as outdated as reality orientation in a few short years, as practitioners realize that the unintended consequences of their efforts produce more harm than good. This iatrogenic effect has led to rethinking the use of restraints and alarms, suppositories and food supplements, and rigid institutional schedules for waking, sleeping, medications, and daily activity.

An area that is now being looked at more carefully is the use of alarms. Alarms don't reduce falls; but they very well may iatrogenically increase the likelihood of an injury from a fall by making residents more brittle as they fear that by moving they will set off the alarm. Consider this: How many new residents in your home fall on their first or second night as they make a trip to the bathroom in the middle of the night? For how many, do you then put on an alarm? This is pretty standard practice in many homes. But the unintended consequence is that alarms often leave a resident more vulnerable to future falls because residents weaken from the inactivity caused by not wanting to set off the alarm. Not only do alarms make matters worse, they also do not address the root cause of the fall—the resident's need for safe passage to the bathroom. The time spent documenting a fall, and responding to alarms that go off each time a resident adjusts her position in bed, is not time well spent, compared to the time taken to make adjustments to prevent someone from falling in the first place by lowering the bed and providing means for a resident to steady herself on the way to the bathroom.

Suppositories and alarms can be iatrogenic in that they cause further decline in a resident's ability to move her bowels or maintain balance and mobility. OBRA '87 addresses iatrogenic decline in its requirement that nursing homes "*attain or maintain* the highest practicable physical, mental, and psychosocial well-being of each resident." The word *practicable* is so unused in common language that it seems like a typo, but it has a very specific meaning and was intentionally used by the authors of OBRA, rather than the word *practical*. While practical means within the limits of the organization, practicable means within the limits of the individual. The surveyor guidelines explain that no one should decline unless the decline is an unavoidable, natural result of a resident's condition. The standard of practice is to prevent or minimize decline and, where possible, help people regain abilities. For residents who are vulnerable to falls, a new approach includes interventions to strengthen their balance, gait, and mobility and make their environment easier to navigate by using trial runs to figure out how to help them make it safely.

Individualized Care is Better Care

Individualized care *is* better care and it is what consumers want. In a landmark study in 1985, The Consumer Perspective on Quality Care: The Residents' Point of View, by the National Citizens Coalition for Nursing Home Reform, several hundred residents talked about what mattered most to them in their daily nursing home life. Their consensus was that kind, caring staff who know them as individuals and accommodate their individual ways of living was the most important factor in the quality of their experience. Decades later, it is still what consumers want. Consumers gravitate toward homes delivering individualized care. The typical consumer cannot express why it is different at this nursing home. They can just feel that it is better. While people still say they would rather die than go to a nursing home, even that is changing as nursing homes learn how to provide a better environment for care and life.

With this evolution, a critical mass of practitioners have already paved the way for the rest of the long-term care field. The federal government, through surveyor guidelines, the survey process, and the

MDS, now emphasizes quality of life as a key means to achieve good care outcomes. One surveyor involved in an Individualized Care Pilot in Rhode Island described how her understanding of good care has evolved:

> One of the things that I thought I was expected to do was to make sure that residents were up and dressed even if it was early in the morning, and having a sigh of relief if they were, thinking we should be having a good survey. Now, I see things very differently. The resident doesn't need to be up until he or she is ready to get up. That starts their whole day in a more favorable way for them.

Now, doing things the way they've always been done is no longer good enough to meet the new and different expectations at every juncture. Change is no longer optional, but necessary for organizations that want to remain viable.

Yet for many organizations, these changes are daunting to the point of feeling unrealistic because living with the stress created by maintaining the institutional patterns actually makes it hard to free up time for rethinking processes of care. In the hectic pace of daily life in traditional nursing homes, staff rush to complete their assignments and routines and to address the problems those institutional routines have iatrogenically caused. Waking people out of a sound sleep to do a two-hour check at night, even for people who never need to be changed at that time, causes sleep deprivation that has a negative effect on residents, which staff spend time addressing all day long.

Homes that have transitioned from institutional schedules to individualized schedules for waking, sleeping, eating, bathing, and other daily activities have seen benefits for residents, staff, and their organization as a whole. Positive results include better nutrition, less plate waste, fewer supplements, fewer suppositories, better clinical outcomes, better resident, family, and staff satisfaction, and less stress. Such changes bring better census, better revenue, and a better bottom line.

Individualized care and staff stability led to aggregate clinical, survey, and financial improvements among the 254 nursing homes that participated in Improving the Nursing Home Culture, the CMS-sponsored pilot conducted by Quality Partners of Rhode Island in 2004–2005. The evidence is in—changing to individualized care gets better results. These evidence-based individualized care practices are now firmly established as the standard of practice. In homes that have individualized their nighttime and morning routines and concentrated on ensuring that residents have a good night's sleep, residents come into the day in a more relaxed way. Even the housekeeping staff notices it. Fewer medications are needed for treating what had been the resident's "environmentally induced" agitation and anxiety. Making changes to engage staff and individualize care will help you reduce iatrogenically caused declines in residents' conditions.

Here are some other areas that are giving nursing homes a lot of traction in their change process:

- To individualize medication administration, the ideal practice is regular review of the medication regimens by a prescribing physician with the pharmacist and with nurses on the unit to make adjustments that accommodate both residents' individual schedules and nursing workflow.

- Best practice in nursing homes is a liberalized diet. Many homes are reducing their number of diets to a mere handful. Having too many diets inhibits the flexibility of food service and the palatability of food. When residents want food that isn't on their diet, they find ways to get it secretly. When what they eat is not fully known, it can't be mitigated. The goal should be to widen the range of what people can eat and use effective mechanisms to manage the impact of what people eat, instead of imposing stringent and unrealistic restrictions.

- The federal government has issued guidance on activities emphasizing individualized activities over group activities, and expecting activities to play a role in nonpharmacological interventions to alleviate psychosocial concerns. The activities staff need to individualize activities for residents and use activities as a way to build relationships among residents.

- There is increasing attention to the first 24 to 48 hours of a resident's stay as a critical period for getting the stay off to a good start. Here is a ripe opportunity for social work services staff to coordinate with unit-based staff in getting to know new residents and helping them settle in. Learning their social history and their daily routines will be as important to unit staff as it is to social work staff. Doing so in tandem will allow social work and CNA/

nursing staff to collaborate in welcoming new residents, ensuring continuity of their personal daily rhythms, and helping them through times when they need psychosocial interventions.

- Coordination between rehabilitation services and unit-based staff is another important best practice. Therapy's usefulness is extended by such coordination. Scheduling of appointments and continuation of rehabilitative activity depend on close partnership. Partnerships are two-way streets in which rehab staff and unit staff work closely to figure out what residents need and to make sure they get it. Collaboration should include contingency plans and flexibility so that residents get their regular therapy without being hampered by rigid schedules that are often unrealistic in the daily flow of life on a unit.

Moving the flywheel is a continual process. Start where you can gather momentum through small changes that have a positive impact. Focus in on areas that reduce stress, stabilize staffing, and build a positive chain of leadership. Use each change as a building block that gives you a foundation for taking on further changes.

Whether you are looking to change care delivery systems or workplace practices, a high-involvement process will get you the best results. Build people's capacity to take on change by engaging staff in identifying what needs to be focused on and how to take it on. As staff see their input used and that the changes produce positive benefits, they will become more engaged. Develop staff's critical thinking skills and the systems that draw them out.

Put infrastructures in place to support day-to-day relational coordination. When staff are used to thinking things through together as part of their routine way of working, they will be more able and eager to contribute to the creative analytical thinking you need from them to succeed in making innovations. Build pillars for collaboration into daily functions—change of shift, start and end of shift stand-up, the care planning process, and quality improvement efforts. Having these key mechanisms for communication in place gives you a foundation for collaboration to make changes.

One good change leads to another. Each change that is put in place and grounded in your policies and practices becomes foundational for the next change. It is the combination of changes, and the growing ability of staff to work together that gets your organization to perform at its best. Long-term care is continually changing. If your organization is nimble and cohesive, you can continually take up opportunities for improvement and lead in pioneering the changes. Once you've got the flywheel moving in a positive cycle, you can take on any change.

## CHAPTER 8

Memo to Corporate

From: David Farrell

I HAVE A NEW PERSPECTIVE. As a 20-year veteran of corporate environments, I've experienced both effective and ineffective regional directors of operations and other nursing home consultants. It was easier to have my opinions of what I'd have liked them to do differently when I was an administrator than it is now that I am a relatively new regional director of operations (6 months) with oversight of nine skilled nursing facilities. Some might say . . . a neophyte.

From my limited experience, I've already learned so much both from the times I've been effective and the times I've been ineffective. I realize now how much what I do in this regional role really matters. As I look at this regional role with fresh eyes, I am not yet sure what *to do*, but I have a pretty clear idea of what I *shouldn't do*.

My leadership wake-up call is that change needs to start with me and how I carry out my role as a corporate regional consultant who visits and oversees nursing homes. As we change our whole approach to teaching and consulting and our long-held ways of communicating with administrators, directors of nursing (DONs), and the department managers, we'll be able to realign our measures and our incentives, on our way from good to great. I've been privileged to see the benefits of this approach and they are compelling.

The first step is to assess how well what we're doing is working, go with what works best, and shed the rest. Borrowing from Jim Collins in *Good to Great*, let's map out our list of things we need to stop doing. Here I also share some ways of doing it differently.

The Stop-Doing List

"Drive-by" Consulting

A common approach taken by corporate regional consultants seems to be one that values the quantity of facility visits over the quality of those consulting visits. The goal seems to be to get to as many facilities as possible every month. And, of course, the most troubled homes get more visits by more consultants. High-performing homes get short, friendly, "rubber stamp" visits. And the low performers receive longer, unfriendly, inspection-type visits. In both cases, and in many instances, these visits are just not very effective, as evidenced by the data remaining the same.

It is certainly not the regional staff's fault. The goal of *volume* of visits has been a long-standing goal of corporate consultants, so they try to achieve that goal. But doing so minimizes their effect. When a regional director has ten homes to consult with and four are troubled (not uncommon in a typical region) there is simply not enough time to effectively influence the troubled homes and the nursing homes functioning well. Maybe the very structure of the regional positions is flawed. Could this emphasis on volume of visits over quality of visits be one of the root causes of why we always have four troubled homes out of ten in the regions?

A better approach to effectively influence a troubled home is to simply park yourself there. Go there every day, consistently, until all the "right people are on the bus, the wrong people are off the bus, and the right people are in the right seats," so the flywheel is spinning toward quality.

It may take 3 months, and you may not get to all ten of the facilities under your watch each week, because you are taking the time necessary to get this one home *right*. We all know the cycle of low performance to minimum compliance and then back to low performance. When we see this pattern, it is a sure sign that our interventions failed. We, the regional consultants, never addressed the root causes of the home's issues because we never took the necessary time to "peel the onion" and get to the core issues that are holding them back.

You simply cannot rush the process of a comprehensive organizational assessment, and the implementation of targeted interventions, which only come from spending time at a place day after day. As issues arise, you discover the barriers and help the team to overcome those people, equipment, and system flaws that are the root of the problem. As you intervene, you teach the facility leadership team how to make changes together and support them as they see the changes work. When you're there mentoring every day, you can build the facility leadership team's capacity to sustain the changes that led to the improvements and avoid the common slide backward that can occur after the regional and corporate staff leave. Regional and corporate staff are only effective in influencing long-term sustained improvement when they teach the entire facility leadership team not simply to follow by rote the new changes in policies and procedures, but also how to work together.

Overlooking Low Staff Satisfaction

Corporate and regional consultants frequently look at the overtime, turnover, and hours per patient per day (PPD). These are three important measures.

On the other hand, staff satisfaction is a key performance measure that has a strong correlation to everything else we are trying to achieve. Yet it is often overlooked.

We have ample research-based evidence to support the fact that staff satisfaction drives employee engagement. And engaged employees is the key to quality. Unhappy staff will derail any attempts to propel an organization to the next level in care and service. Yet most regional and corporate staff are focused somewhere else. The truth is, we, the corporate staff, need to give our administrators, DONs, and department managers, including charge nurses, the tools, training, and budget to show the frontline staff that we care about them and their job stress, and we will listen to them. And the hard truth is we, the corporate staff, need to learn how to do it ourselves and begin to treat the nursing home leaders in such a way as to drive up their satisfaction and engagement. Maybe our behavior and communication style help drive high turnover of administrators and DONs, who burn out as fast as the certified nursing assistants (CNAs) and licensed vocational nurses (LVNs).

Dr. V. Tellis-Nayak has done some excellent research regarding the feelings and perceptions of administrators and DONs. Tellis-Nayak asked them about us, nursing home corporate and regional staff, and the results are not pretty. It was evident that we de-motivate administrators and DONs yet expect them to motivate their staff.

If we focus only on short-term outcome measures of overtime, turnover, and hours PPD, we end up forcing administrators and DONs to focus on the outcomes instead of the key process measures that drive those outcomes—the data from employee satisfaction reports. As a result, the managers implement ineffective solutions that don't address the root cause. Instead, the misguided efforts and action plans often contribute to turnover, burnout, stress, more unscheduled absences, and low morale.

As regional consultants, we need to help administrators and DONs boost morale, engage their staff, and stabilize staffing and schedules, even if it means extra hours PPD in the short run. In the long run, when staff can count on consistent and fair leadership and scheduling, they experience daily stability in their work and, in turn, are reliable and consistent in their performance.

Educating only the Administrators and DONs

A fundamental flaw in our approach to help trigger improvement in nursing homes is our reliance on educating only the administrators and DONs and then expecting them to take the information back to their facility and effectively implement it or share it with their staff. It does not work. Education of only two leaders is definitely a burden to the leaders. Unfortunately, most of the information dumped on administrators and DONs at the typical monthly meeting rarely gets back to the staff who need it most—especially when it comes to the way the organization will move forward with person-centered care changes. That is primarily because it is as much about the process of change as it is the changes themselves. Leaders don't succeed through policy changes and strict mandates. They succeed by engaging staff in understanding why something is important and in figuring out how to make it work.

Our new corporate educational mantra needs to be "educate all facility staff instead of two individual facility leaders." And the education, coaching, and mentoring are best done on the leaders' and staff's home turf, with their unique issues and barriers, personalities and communication styles. In that way, we model the process that we want the leaders to provide their staff: hands-on, ground-up, collaborative problem solving.

Retaining Consultants without a Process to Monitor and Improve Their Performance

There are some key questions to ask. How well do we seek the feedback from the nursing home leaders that we are consulting with? Do we ever ask the administrators and DONs how effective our consultants are? Do our consultants get the honest feedback and coaching *they* need to be better consultants? Do we educate our corporate and regional consultants on how to be more effective in the consulting role?

Let's be honest—it is rare to find a long-term care (LTC) company doing any of this. Our customers (the administrators, DONs, and department managers) are left without a voice when it comes to feedback regarding the people consulting and supervising them. As a result, ineffective LTC leaders and consultants can stay in their job for years, while doing it quite ineffectively, according to the ones they are educating, supervising, and consulting with. If a home is cycling in and out of compliance, it is a sure sign that the corporate consultation isn't working; yet often it is the administrators and DONs who lose their jobs, while the corporate team just goes on in the same manner, with their same toolkit, with the next crop of leaders. Compliance problems usually have both people and systemic causes, and until those causes are fixed, the problems will remain.

When there are problems, corporate consultants need to get to work with the leadership to build the capacity for root cause analysis and customized interventions. Often, instead, we come in with a rote simplistic plan—our policies, training on those policies, and monitoring of those policies. When the policies are developed without a true process of understanding the underlying causes and working together to develop solutions that will be operational for the long term, then we merely put in place the temporary fix needed to pass resurvey. But staff can't sustain policies imposed from the outside that make no sense in their daily operations. The policies may have a process that simply does not make sense for that particular home. Then it needs slight adjusting to fit. But, without taking the time to adjust that process, the policy adds one more stress as the pitfall remains. Then the home is more vulnerable next time because the problems have resurfaced.

Let's change this ineffective practice and start by hiring experts to help educate our regional staff and corporate consultants to be more effective consultants and teachers. We need to learn to take a capacity-building approach to our interventions. We need to measure our success as corporate staff by the facility leadership's ability to solve their own problems with our coaching. Rather than cut off thinking, we need to help the frontline leaders use their critical thinking skills to develop customized solutions that will work in their buildings.

Next, let's allow the facility leaders to rate the effectiveness of their supervisors and consultants on a quarterly basis. Let's ask facility leaders how well their supervisors and consultants are helping them be better leaders and bringing out the critical thinking skills in their staff. This *internal customer* feedback is just the kind of information needed to trigger the self-reflection necessary to turn around an ineffective corporate or regional executive.

Finally, let's also self-reflect on our own effectiveness and ask ourselves some simple questions: How effective am I? What is my influence on the nursing homes I consult with? How do the leaders and staff respond to me? Am I a mentor and a coach and a teacher or am I an inspector and a criticizer and a de-motivator? Do the structural, procedural, or outcome measures improve as a result of my consultation? What can I do better next time to increase my effectiveness as a consultant?

Ignoring the Best Performers

There are some incredible leaders in the LTC profession—administrators, DONs, department managers, and caregivers who do amazing things every day. Yet, we spend most of our time in the lower-performing homes and only give the high performers a call when the census dips or an issue rises to the corporate level. This de-motivates people. We should, as regional staff and corporate executives, be reminding the best performers more consistently how much we appreciate their solid, steady performance.

They need more on-site visits from us with specific praise as we observe their excellent practices in action. They need a call just to say, "I appreciate all you are doing there. Thank you very much. We do not take your commitment lightly."

Most corporate nursing home executives and regional staff reading this are going to say, "I do that." But are you sure? Then why are so many high-performing administrators and DONs so unhappy? At the regional and corporate level, we all can't be doing a great job of this. Tellis-Nayak's research data simply do not support our view of how much praise we offer our administrators and DONs. We need to do more. We need to be more effective at putting these people, with all the power, at their "best" every day.

Ken Blanchard, in *The One Minute Manager*, says that praise needs to be "timely, specific, sincere, proportional, and positive." As regional staff, we tend to call administrators about problems—census, costs, and deficiencies. If they're doing a good job, they might not even be on the list for needing a call because their census is up, their costs and deficiencies are down. It is very discouraging for high performers to hear from us primarily when we need them to cut their food costs, even if we do say in the call that we appreciate the high occupancy rates they are achieving. Let's stop and ask, is the food really good? What do the satisfaction surveys say? What is their pressure sore rate? How is the resident weight loss there? Just maybe, the higher *investment* in the food is a key contributing factor of other successful outcomes.

Instead of nitpicking on an expense line item or two, let's call our high performers on a regular basis to let leaders know their numbers are looking good and to ask what help they need. And ask how you can help them achieve excellence in the next area they are focused on. Even more important, ask for more information about what they're doing that is working so well. Lead them in a root cause analysis of something that they are highly successful at. Then use their identified root causes of the good outcomes to help other facility leaders with the specifics they need to help them improve.

Let the good leaders know you see them and value them. If they are doing well 90% of the time, you need to make sure 90% of your communication with them is proportionally positive.

In my current job, when we received our staff satisfaction data and realized we needed to improve, we set up learning collaboratives that were focused on employee relations. The collaboratives were structured after the Institute for Healthcare Improvement's (IHI) collaborative model, which is designed to improve clinical outcomes among a group of healthcare providers. The collaborative learning sessions were a perfect way for our best performers to share what they do well in a way that helped everyone else improve. Bringing leaders together to spread good practice acknowledges your strong performers in a way that lets them know you see what they're doing and appreciate it so much you want others to follow their lead.

Treating Administrators Like "Gofers"

One of administrators' biggest frustrations is being trusted with the health and welfare of 110 residents 365 days a year with oversight of a multimillion-dollar budget yet having to ask for approval to give an employee a raise 1% over the standard. As an administrator, you often feel second-guessed by regional staff and corporate executives who do not have all the information. You feel guilty, like you need to prove your innocence to the people who are supposed to be on your side. And you receive stinging emails that can leave you wondering if anyone cares but you.

We have created a policy and procedure for everything and a workforce of gofers instead of LTC leaders with an entrepreneurial spirit. Certainly, the Department of Health Services and their enforcement practices have contributed to this malaise. After all, achieving the minimum standard is the goal for many leaders. But, once again, how about us? Do we treat them like we want them to follow the policies and procedures instead of thinking and acting like a leader and like an owner.

Some Administrators and DONs get so demoralized that they are sometimes just "punching the clock." They have lost all sense of being able to have an impact, and so they do not act like they care. In their hearts, they still care. Yet the staff perceives their leader's outside appearance and words as a lack of caring. Data from My InnerView (an independent, applied research company that measures satisfaction of residents, family members, and staff in over 6,000 nursing homes nationwide) finds that our greatest opportunity to impact our employees' overall satisfaction at work is to improve their perception of how well their leaders care about them.

Most facility leaders come to this work with a desire to make a difference and a willingness to work hard to do so. Corporate and regional consultants have an obligation to nurture that spirit, not crush it. For those who are worn out and just doing their time, we need to give them honest feedback and collect the data (staff satisfaction survey data) of staff perceptions that reveal the "brutal facts." But again, how much do our current approaches with these nursing home leaders contribute to their uncaring approach with their own staff.

Simply put, how corporate and regional consultants treat facility leaders directly affects how the facility leaders treat their own staff. Of course, facility staff will treat the residents as they are treated by the facility leaders.

Focusing on Policies Instead of People

Administrators and DONs have an enormous impact on the performance of nursing homes. Their leadership practices and daily actions influence all the outcomes that a nursing home is getting. Yet regional and corporate staff tend to lean toward checking compliance with policies rather than focusing on the leaders and what they are doing that is not producing the desired results. We lean toward chart audits instead of organizational and leadership assessments.

Clearly, it is much easier to check compliance with policies as opposed to dealing with giving an administrator the honest feedback that he or she needs to perform better this afternoon. Checking charts and writing reports about the findings are important but should not be the primary tasks of the facility visit. Consulting visits should always include some feedback of leaders' performance. If it does not appear that thorough rounds were done, say so. If staff is avoiding eye contact with the boss during rounds, ask why. If no one is smiling, express concern. If meetings are held without group process, and the administrator or DON is the only one speaking, teach them a better way.

On the other hand, if you observe an exemplary LTC leader who is saying and doing all the right things and clearly has engaged the staff, articulate your observations regarding the leader's effectiveness so that the person continues those actions.

An organization steeped in rules and compliance with policies will not be able to adapt to changing circumstances or the many unexpected situations that routinely occur in a people-oriented operation. Most circumstances that arise in nursing homes require the staff to problem solve together. Ultimately, the leaders who help people work well together will be more effective than the leaders who focus strictly on adherence to rigid rules. Leaders who do regular teamwork-oriented rounds and have their finger on the pulse of the building know what circumstances their staff are dealing with and can use on-the-spot teachable moments to problem solve together. It is this ability to huddle and problem solve that makes an organization agile, resilient, and effective in handling any situation that comes its way. It positions the organization to be person centered. It triggers high-quality care and service.

Using the Wrong Measures to Assess Leadership

Department of Health inspection results and executing a complex budget are two important measures of the effectiveness of administrators and DONs. However, these outcome measures are the end result of many critical structural and procedural measures.

Key quality process measures such as staff satisfaction, resident satisfaction, and family members satisfaction are important measures of LTC leadership performance for their own sake and they have been proven by Tellis-Nayak, Leslie Grant, and My InnerView to be proxies for solid and sustained performance over the long term. Structural measures of quality that lead to satisfaction, such as staff stability, staffing consistency, and employee absenteeism, should also be used to judge administrators' and DONs' performance. Poor outcomes in these process and structural measures of quality often result in poor inspection results and underwhelming financial performance. Therefore, LTC administrators and DONs, as well as regional consultants and their corporate executives, should all be carefully collecting data and assessing performance in the quality metrics with the strongest influence on the outcomes. By focusing everyone here, we have the greatest likelihood to positively affect the overall organization and its performance.

If we don't take these measures seriously, and respond only to outcomes such as financial or survey results, we often send facilities down a path that starts a vicious cycle with continued declines. If the facility is over budget and the response from corporate is to cut food costs, or positions, without understanding the root cause of the issues, it will likely lead to more turnover, call-offs, and overtime, as well as disgruntled residents and family members. The cuts then lead to lower performance, lower census, and a financial loss.

By focusing on staff, resident, and family satisfaction, the facility will reduce turnover and unscheduled absences, which will reduce overtime, agency, and other associated staffing costs. It is better to spend smart, where every staffing dollar contributes positively to stability, rather than to be "penny-wise and pound foolish." Similarly, stabilizing staffing is the first step in addressing any quality concerns or survey issues. When staffing is unstable, residents get inconsistent, rushed, harried, depersonalized care by stressed-out staff.

When staffing stabilizes, everyone feels the benefit, and outcomes improve.

Ignoring the Obligation to Lower Staff Stressors

Stress puts our staff at their worst. Stressed-out staff make errors, use poor judgment, skip crucial steps in a policy, and tend to snap at one another and at the residents. My InnerView finds that LTC leaders' lack of focus on lowering work-related stress is a major contributor to lower overall satisfaction on the job. Unfortunately, important meetings among the corporate and regional staff rarely have an agenda item devoted to this issue of reducing staff stress. Staff stress is simply not on our radar screen.

It is time to change that focus. Not only do we need to do a better job of both monitoring and assessing the causes of employee stress, we need to teach administrators and DONs to do the same. Most LTC leaders can quickly identify the stressors for the staff. Yet they do not seem to devote much energy to overcoming the stressors for the front-line staff.

Within the book, we offer many insights into staff stressors and how to mitigate them. Of course, staff instability is the biggest stressor of all. As corporate and regional consultants, we need to accept that until a facility's staffing is stabilized, consistent assignment is in place, and morale is up, improvement in any other areas will be unlikely or short lived.

To relieve staff stressors we need to make sure staff have the following:

- The equipment and supplies they need to do their job

- Hours and schedules they can count on

- Employee assistance programs to tap into when life off the job presents problems that affect their performance on the job

- Ways to provide for their health and the health of their families. (With the high cost of health insurance, think about ways of providing some health benefits—free flu shots; smoking cessation and weight loss programs; healthy snacks in the vending machine; healthy low-cost food for free or for purchase.)

Some stressors are caused by poor supervision, or by work practices that make the workload too hard and force staff to cut corners just to get the basics done. We have an obligation to make sure staff work for good supervisors and that we examine the flow of work to remove any burdens that get in the way of their ability to do their job in a high-quality, person-centered way.

Failing to Budget Enough Funds to Engage Staff

LTC organizations need to constantly invest in an evidence-based approach to create and/or sustain engaged employees. Therefore, it is wise for corporate to budget the dollars to invest in staff engagement and, regardless of the current profitability and occupancy rates, encourage the administrator and DON to spend that money consistently yet wisely.

It is also critical for regional consultants to teach LTC leaders how to make wise investments with these budgeted funds. For example, a DON can choose to spend $350 and feed all the staff pizza by putting it in the break room. People are told that the pizza is a big "thank you" from administration to staff. The employees on all three shifts are fed, and the leadership feels good that they bought the pizza. They believe, "we improved morale." Well . . . maybe, maybe not.

Alternatively, the DON may choose to invest that same $350 in a way that is more likely to spark the staff to perform even better. For example, the DON notes a significant decline in resident falls with injuries. So she goes out and buys $100 worth of Popsicles and spends $250 on nine gifts at Cost Plus World Market. She buys three jewelry boxes, three boxes of dinner plates, two framed pictures, and a box of wine glasses. That afternoon, the DON calls a quick neighborhood meeting within each neighborhood and shares the improved resident fall data and the Popsicles and then raffles off two of the gifts to the individuals in attendance on the neighborhood. She acknowledges the staff's efforts to keep the residents safe and outlines the key resident safety approaches that are helping to reduce falls. The DON repeats these meetings on each neighborhood on each different shift.

As you can see, it is the same dollar investment in both examples, yet the second scenario will more likely create the staff engagement needed both to sustain the gains made with fall prevention and to get the staff energized to take on the next challenge. In the second case, the DON creates excitement by saying, "Timeout, look at these data. See? We are winning! And you are making it happen. Let's review what we are doing to make this happen. Isn't this exciting!"

At the corporate and regional level, we would be wise to provide both the budget and the direction regarding how to "invest" budgeted funds to engage the staff. Let's spend less on pizza and more on true "carrots."

Going Cheap on Products for Residents and Staff

The quality of the toilet paper, paper towels, hand soap, body soap, shampoo, linens, and resident trash bags is noticed by the staff and residents who use them the most. Cheap products affect outcomes in an environment where the end user of those products is the fragile skin of nursing home residents.

Cheap products can also create inefficiencies and increase costs. For example, purchasing cheap trash bags for the resident rooms may appear to save money at first glance. But if both the housekeepers and the CNAs have to double bag everything due to their experience with the cheap bags breaking, then the cost savings is eliminated. It actually costs more when you factor in the inefficiencies and labor costs associated with frustrated staff who have to take extra time to double bag everything.

Going cheap on everything sends a loud message: "We don't care." The frontline staff perceives that the purchase of these low-quality products means that saving money is more important than people. In no way are we advocating for fiscal irresponsibility. But let's not be so cheap. In other words, it does not have to be "pillow-soft Charmin," but it does need to be two-ply.

Conducting Traditional Corporate/Regional Meetings versus Learning Sessions

One model that was highly effective in spreading both clinical and leadership best practices was tested across thousands of nursing homes nationwide as part of the CMS Nursing Home Quality Initiative. State quality improvement organizations adopted and adapted the Institute for Healthcare Improvement's Breakthrough Series Collaborative Model, which is designed to spread evidence-based clinical, organizational culture change and leadership best practices. Providers responded with measurable clinical, workforce, survey, and financial gains across a broad base of measures. While there can be very strict methods to the Institute for Healthcare Improvement (IHI) approach, doing IHI "lite" works just as well in promoting sharing among leaders of homes in a corporation. When the IHI collaborative approach is used, the typically dry administrator and director of nursing meeting shifts away from being a top-down transmittal of information to a learning session that is organized in a way that facilitates the sharing of ideas and challenges among all participants. Collaborative learning sessions include education that can help with key challenges and time for discussion of the practical applications of the information. When people come together at the next learning session, they share what they have done and learned, and where they still need help to take their improvements further.

If nursing home corporations and regional teams were to adopt some of the key components contained within the IHI collaborative model, significant and sustained improvement would be a much more realistic goal. The added bonus is that the IHI model taps into the collective wisdom of the entire group of attendees: *everybody teaches, and everybody learns.* As a result, the leaders who attend the learning session become engaged through group process exercises, presenting their experience initiating similar changes and learning from others who are initiating change at their nursing home.

Learning sessions become just that: a meeting during which leaders learn and then initiate change. Administrators and their teams of change agents come to learning sessions prepared to present what they changed based on what they learned from the preceding meeting. The peer-to-peer exchange of core, foundational implementation steps helps fuel the others to make changes as well.

The IHI collaborative model triggers the administrator to make change because of the following:

- The team from his or her nursing home is in attendance with him or her.

- The team has time to plan changes with the administrator during the learning session.

- The team has to present to the other participants what they changed and what happened as a result at each learning session. Thus, there is healthy peer pressure to make changes and present well at the learning sessions. As a result, there is a greater likelihood that changes will actually occur back at the nursing home after learning sessions.

Thinking that Traditional Bonus Plans Motivate Facility Leaders

The highest-performing administrators and DONs rarely think about the bonus. It is not a daily motivator. Yet, some corporate executives and regional staff, who are highly motivated by their quarterly or annual bonus (which is largely dependent on the performance of the administrators and DONs), assume that these high performers have the same motivation for the bonus as they do. They openly discuss the bonus with the high-performing administrators and DONs without realizing that, in many cases, the focus on the bonus by the corporate and regional staff can actually turn off the facility leaders.

It is more effective to tap into these facility leaders' intrinsic motivators, which are often associated with resident and family members' praise, their staff's accomplishments, clinical outcomes, progress toward person-centered care, and human resource outcomes, including employee satisfaction and retention.

Without a doubt, they like the bonus dollars, and they regularly achieve the bonus, but it is not a motivator. You may even consider that their lack of focus on the bonus allows them to be so successful. We are likely to increase our effectiveness as corporate and regional consultants if we focus less on the bonus plans and more on treating the administrators and DONs as individuals and then taking the time to understand their motivators and acting on the information.

A better way is to start by basing 50% of the bonus dollars on resident, family member, and staff satisfaction survey response rates and scores. Next, let's include some bonus dollars on the key measures of stability: consistent assignment, absenteeism, and turnover rates. Finally, how about quarterly bonus payouts for achieving minimal resident falls and an in-house-acquired pressure ulcer rate below 2%.

Disregarding Staffing Coordinators

No one is more powerful than the staffing coordinators. Yet the regional and corporate executives often ignore this key individual. The staffing coordinator often holds all the answers, but the administrator and the DON are often asked all the questions.

Let's start focusing our attention on this key person, the staffing coordinator, and the wealth of knowledge and information that he or she can offer. Regional and corporate staff should always connect directly with this individual on each visit and include him or her in the discussions regarding staff stability and consistent assignment.

We would serve our staff and residents well by carefully examining the staffing books, schedules, and assignment sheets. We are looking for well-organized staffing books, schedules that are posted well in advance, staff assignment sheets with few written deletions, and evidence of the consistency of the licensed staff and CNA assignments. Asking the staffing coordinator about call-outs, open positions, consistent assignments, and other important staffing issues ensures the regional staff will get valid information. Coach this person while you examine the schedules together. Assess the composition of the staff by counting how many part-time staff are being assigned shifts each day compared to full-time staff. Investment of the regional consultants' time in educating our staffing coordinators can have a strong, positive impact on organizational performance.

Assessing LTC Leadership Based Solely on State Survey Inspection Results

Some outstanding leaders running excellent homes receive a level "G" deficiency, and some weak LTC leaders managing marginal homes have deficiency-free surveys. Bad things can happen under excellent leaders, and good things can happen under the watch of weak leaders in LTC. Therefore, we should incorporate a broad base of key performance measures of LTC leaders and rely less on an outcome measure that, when taken alone, is a flawed measure of quality in LTC according to researchers.

We have more accurate and reliable measures of LTC leadership performance that have already been outlined here—for instance, simply no one is a better judge of leadership performance than the residents, their families, and the staff, whose input can be obtained through the distribution and collection of anonymous satisfaction surveys. Administrators, DONs, and their department managers should be assessed using satisfaction data, human resource outcomes, and clinical quality measures. State survey inspection results, while important, should not be the ultimate measure of performance.

Retaining Low-performing Staff

We have very little technology in nursing homes and no machinery producing something. It is all people. People matter most. Human beings drive nursing home organizational performance. In nursing homes, the people who work there are producing the outcomes you are getting and the reputation that you have. A nursing home is never great without a lot of great people working there.

It is true that policies and procedures that drive systems, as well as equipment and supplies, are important. However, it seems that at the regional level, we tend to focus more on the adherence to the policies (systems) as the absolute key to improving quality, and we spend very little time really looking at the people working there or coaching nursing home leadership staff on how to spur better performance.

Let's address the root cause of why low-performing nursing homes stay low performing. They retain the wrong staff. And we (corporate and regional consultants) write action plan after action plan to address major issues, but we fail to focus the leadership team on their low performers, the *people* who are holding them back, and provide them with a comprehensive methodology to make the changes necessary to trigger higher performance. During consultant visits, we may identify the obvious one or two low performers and may ask whether we need to get rid of them. But we often fail to provide the administrator and the DON with a process with which to assess their entire staff and then make the personnel moves necessary to trigger quality improvement and an enhanced reputation that comes with it.

Poor-performing people can keep the whole organization sputtering between *good* and *fair* performance with occasional times of *serious safety risk*. All the oversight and the training in the world can't move the group to the next level because the poor-performing staff affect others' performance in a negative way. These individuals are a compounding force. Thus removing them and replacing them with someone better does not simply improve a small corner of the nursing home; the positive change spreads to others because of the high interdependent nature of the majority of tasks that nursing home employees perform.

Relational competence matters—it matters a lot. Relational competence is the ability to positively relate to others. Staff who have relational competence are people who have excellent communication skills and willingly smile at others. When you combine the addition of someone with relational competence with the removal of staff without relational competence, regardless of skill set, communication and teamwork increase dramatically the next shift. As a result, resident care and service improve.

One comprehensive way for our nursing home leadership teams to assess their staff is to take the following steps:

1. Make a list of all of the most reliable staff based on each employee's attendance record.

2. Meet with the nursing leadership team and, name by name, discuss and then rank individual staff members based on their clinical

skills and their attitude (how they relate to and treat residents and their co-workers). Under both categories (Clinical and Attitude) rank each staff member as either *excellent*, *good*, or *fair*. Allow for some healthy discussion among the team as they discuss and rank each staff member.

3.   When the list is complete, put a star next to the reliable employees with excellent clinical skills and excellent attitudes. These are the Triple Crown winners. These are the employees you cannot afford to lose. They are the reason why you get thank-you cards from grateful family members. And facilities need to employ a comprehensive approach to keep their Triple Crown winners engaged and employed there. Count how many Triple Crown winners you have working there.

4.   Make a list of the unreliable staff and rank their clinical skills and attitude in the same way. Focus on those who are rated as having fair clinical skills and a fair attitude. These are the Triple Crown losers and the employees you cannot afford to keep. They damage the reputation of the facility and put it at risk. Doing nothing and continuing to tolerate their low performance holds back the home from achieving higher quality. Count how many Triple Crown losers you have working there.

5.   Make a plan. Replace the Triple Crown losers with new hires who have the potential to be Triple Crown winners by utilizing an improved method of attracting, selecting, and training new staff (see Chapter 2, Taking Time to Hire Right). The higher the number of Triple Crown winners, the greater the likelihood the home will achieve quality person-centered care.

6.   Focus back on the list of reliable staff. Look for those who have excellent clinical skills but who were ranked as having only a good or fair attitude. Meet with them. Let them know their strengths, and provide these staff members with feedback about the leadership team's observations of a negative attitude. Ask for improvement.

7.   Focus back on the list of unreliable staff. If you find an individuals ranked as having excellent skills and an excellent attitude but their attendance record reflects unreliablility, then meet with them and coach them into being more reliable. After all, if they start showing up for work when scheduled, you will have one more Triple Crown winner.

The longer the low performance of the organization has been sustained and the poorer the reputation, then the higher the likelihood that the lowest-performing 7 to 10 staff members within the organization may need to be replaced by better people. Certainly, as the number of Triple Crown losers replaced by Triple Crown winners increases, the higher the likelihood of seeing a dramatic and sustained improvement across a broad base of performance metrics.

Some leaders believe that in a unionized home they can never dismiss an employee who is a low performer. However, it can be done. First, make your expectations known clearly to everyone. Second, hold people accountable and make sure to do so fairly and across the board. Then, be very attentive and specific about where a low performer is falling short. Sincerely offer supports to help the employee improve and regular feedback about whether or not improvements are taking place. Document everything along the way. If you have good reasons, a fair process, sincere support, and detailed documentation, you can hold people accountable to high performance standards in a union environment.

Remember to focus the nursing home's administrator and director of nursing attention on those staff ranked at the top and at the bottom. Those ranked at the top and the bottom (look at the count) have a strong pull on those ranked in the middle. When poor performance is tolerated, many staff ranked in the middle wear blinders and just focus on their own survival. As you shift the environment, you will find many of the staff ranked in the middle will respond well to the people changes happening around them. They will step up as weak performers are replaced with potential Triple Crown winners. Often, when they see that you will hold everyone accountable by letting go of the staff who are most responsible for a negative environment, they will improve to the new norm.

Spending Too Little Time on Employee Satisfaction

Staff satisfaction survey results provide corporate and regional staff with the roadmap to quality within each of the nursing homes they oversee. These data allow regional and corporate staff to peer in and come to a deeper understanding of how the frontline staff view the nursing home leadership team. Furthermore, it allows for the development of a specific action plan to boost morale and trigger organization-wide improvement. The root cause has to be addressed if we expect the outcomes to improve.

When a corporate and regional team sees a home with very high staff satisfaction scores, they would be wise to invest more there. High staff engagement is very difficult to achieve in LTC. So if a home has it, and the data prove it, the home has the foundational core element to achieve high-quality outcomes. Outcome data may reflect they are not there yet—they are good but not great—but a minor investment in an area that will give them a boost may be all that is needed to get them to the next level. On the other hand, a corporation could make all kinds of investments in a facility with low staff satisfaction and realize only the disappointment of a lower return on that investment and not the outcomes they were hoping for.

Trimming Hours/Shifts of Best-performing Staff

Resident safety and quality of life are at stake every shift, every day. Yet, when the occupancy dips, we tend to focus on being *fair* when it comes to cutting staff hours rather than being *sensible*. We need to stop being fair to individual staff members and start being fair to everyone in the home.

Lives are at stake, so in a low-census situation where you are expected to cut CNA labor hours, nursing home leaders should always give the shifts to their best performers (Triple Crown winners and the next highest ranked). In the nursing home setting, length of employment does not necessarily mean the individual is reliable and delivers high-quality care with a positive attitude. More often than not, nursing home staffing coordinators are using either employee tenure or a rotation model to guide their decision-making process of cutting staff hours during times of low occupancy. When tenure is used, the veteran staff keep their hours. Under the rotation model, all staff take a turn being called off when the census is low. Both of these methods of determining whose hours are cut make no sense. If the goal is to deliver high-quality, person-centered care, then don't cut the hours of the best performing staff and allow the lower performers to work. If you have to trim hours, in the name of quality person-centered care and resident safety, always cut the shifts of the lowest-ranked staff first, regardless of their tenure.

Ignoring the Importance of Conducting Thorough Rounds with Facility Leaders

Thorough rounds should be the priority, and for many corporate and regional consultants it is. However, just as important as the rounds themselves is how the corporate and regional staff behave during the walk-through. It is what they observe and say during the rounds that is the key.

Corporate and regional consultants can trigger a great boost in morale if they take the time to introduce themselves to staff members, ask them key questions, and act genuinely interested in their responses. Noticing all that is going right and delivering well-deserved compliments can go a long way toward ensuring that those behaviors producing the observed outcomes are repeated.

Conducting rounds with the home's leaders helps to model the way. Regional consultants who conduct rounds with the home's leaders and verbalize their observations and actions along the way are employing an excellent way to teach. Corporate and regional staff often harp on the importance of the nursing homes' leaders to conduct rounds. Yet, we often fail to teach how to effectively conduct rounds because we don't go on rounds together.

Taking Calls While Meeting with Facility Staff

Why should regional and corporate consultants travel to consult with a home's leadership team only to spend the majority of their time on the phone or on email with others? If we are on-site at a facility, then we should focus there. We should spend our time and energy on the people in front of us and avoid the pull of other pressing issues in other facilities. That is easy to write here and difficult to do. But it is the only sure way to mitigate future emergency calls and emails from the other facilities. The more time we spend in a facility but are focused on other homes, the less positive influence we have on the one in front of us, and the greater the likelihood that this home will be calling tomorrow with the next crisis when we are at another home.

I've been privileged throughout my career to have worked with regional and corporate staff who have shown me by their example the benefits of real support and guidance. I strive to pass that knowledge forward.

What Are Your Financial Incentives?

Appendixes A and B are sample drill-down tools excerpted from the Staff Stability Toolkit, produced by Quality Partners of Rhode Island. They are available as downloadable Microsoft Excel spreadsheets at www.riqualitypartners.org by clicking on "HATCh" and then "Workforce." These drill-down tools were originally developed by the authors for their work on Achieving Staff Stability for Better Jobs, Better Care–VT (see Chapter 5). David Johnson of IPRO (New York State's QIO) transformed them into user-friendly, customizable spreadsheets for inclusion in the Staff Stability Toolkit.

What are your financial incentives?

Compile information on types of financial incentives available to staff and determine how frequently they are paid.

Examples of frequently used financial incentives: *Enter information ONLY IN the SHADED Cells. All others will be calculated automatically.*

Bonus for accepting last minute assignment

Comments:	$10/hr RNs and LPNs, $5/hr CNAs
How much was spent last quarter?	$90,000.00
Annual $ est. based on quarter expense-	$360,000.00

Differentials

Position	AM/hr	PM/hr	NOC/hr	Wkend/hr	Amt. Paid Last Qtr	Annual Estimate
RN	$0.00	$3.00	$4.00	$0.50	$31,940.00	$127,760.00
LPN	$0.00	$3.00	$4.00	$0.50	$35,730.00	$142,920.00
CNA	$0.00	$2.00	$2.50	$0.50	$36,028.00	$144,112.00
"Other"	$0.00					$0.00
				TOTALS-->	$103,698.00	$414,792.00

Comments: sample comments for differentials

Baylor

(Offering individual who work two 12-hour shifts and are paid for 30-36 hours of work / 6 to 12 hour premium add-on)

Position	Premium Add-On Amount Paid Last Qtr	Annual Estimate	Comments:
RN	$13,572.00	$54,288.00	work 2 12-hour shifts- get paid for 30- (figures represent 6-hour add-on premium)
LPN	$21,801.00	$87,204.00	
CNA	$31,863.00	$127,452.00	
TOTALS	$67,236.00	$268,944.00	

Position	Average Regular Hourly Rate	Calculated Hourly Rate with 6-Hour Add-On Premium	Calculated Hourly Rate with 8-Hour Add-On Premium	Calculated Hourly Rate with 12-Hour Add-On Premium
RN	$29.00	$36.25	$38.67	$43.50
LPN	$21.50	$26.88	$28.67	$32.25
CNA	$10.75	$13.44	$14.33	$16.13

Enter information ONLY IN the SHADED Cells. All others will be calculated automatically.

Comments:

RNs, LPNs, and CNAs- $1/hr

Per Diem Status

(Extra per hour add-on pay for Per Diem status)

Position	Amt. Paid Last Qtr	Annual Estimate
RN	$6,552.00	$26,208.00
LPN	$2,886.00	$11,544.00
CNA	$3,315.00	$13,260.00
"Other"		$0.00
TOTALS	$12,753.00	$51,012.00

Perfect Attendance Bonus

(No call-outs for a month or quarter)

Position	Amt. Paid Last Qtr	Annual Estimate
RN	$0.00	$0.00
LPN	$0.00	$0.00
CNA	$0.00	$0.00
"Other"	$0.00	$0.00
TOTALS	$0.00	$0.00

Holiday Bonus

(Extra pay for working the holiday above the standard "time and a half")

Position	Amt. Paid Last Qtr	Annual Estimate	Comments:
RN	$0.00	$0.00	
LPN	$0.00	$0.00	
CNA	$0.00	$0.00	
"Other"	$0.00	$0.00	
TOTALS	$0.00	$0.00	

New Employee "Sign On" Bonus

Position	Amt. Paid Last Qtr	Annual Estimate	Comments:
RN	$8,000.00	$32,000.00	RN $2,000;LPN $500;CNA $250;(payout at 6 months)
LPN	$2,000.00	$8,000.00	
CNA	$2,500.00	$10,000.00	
"Other"		$0.00	
TOTALS	$12,500.00	$50,000.00	

Enter information ONLY IN the SHADED Cells. All others will be calculated automatically.

SUMMARY OF BONUSES, INCENTIVES, DIFFERENTIALS AND WAGE INCREASE DATA

Category	Annualized Amount	Comments (auto-filled from worksheet)
Bonus for accepting last minute assignment	$360,000.00	$10/hr RNs and LPNs, $5/hr CNAs
Differentials	$414,792.00	sample comments for differentials
Baylor	$288,944.00	work 2 12-hour shifts- get paid for 30- (figures represent 8-hour add-on premium)
Per Diem Status	$51,012.00	RNs, LPNs, and CNAs- $1/hr
Perfect Attendance Bonus	$0.00	I am trying to figure out what happens if there are more characters than can usually fit in a box of this size... does the text wrap and make the cell larger or not.
Holiday Bonus	$0.00	
New Employee "Sign On" Bonus	$50,000.00	RN $2,000,LPN $500, CNA $250.(payout at 6 months)
Employee "Referral" Bonus	$6,000.00	RN- $1000, LPN- $1000,CNA- $500.(payout at 6 months)
Longevity Bonus	$0.00	
Preceptor Bonus- CNA	$0.00	CNA $300 plus .50/hour
Enter Name of Incentive Program Here	$0.00	test again in the category
Enter Name of Incentive Program Here	$0.00	
Enter Name of Incentive Program Here	$60.00	
Enter Name of Incentive Program Here	$48.00	
Enter Name of Incentive Program Here	$8.00	test
TOTAL ANNUAL ESTIMATE OF ALL BONUSES, INCENTIVES, AND DIFFERENTIALS-	$1,150,864.00	
TOTAL ANNUAL WAGE INCREASE EXPENSE (RNs, LPNs AND CNAs ONLY)-	$90,710.00	

Built on work developed by David Farrell, Quality Partners of Rhode Island, with Cathie Brady and Barbara Frank of B&F Consulting, under contract with Better Jobs Better Care - Vermont.

This material was prepared by IPRO, the Medicare Quality Improvement Organization for New York State, under contract with the Centers for Medicare & Medicaid Services (CMS), an agency of the U.S. Department of Health and Human Services. The contents presented do not necessarily reflect CMS policy.

Tracking Absenteeism

Appendixes A and B are sample drill-down tools excerpted from the Staff Stability Toolkit, produced by Quality Partners of Rhode Island. They are available as downloadable Microsoft Excel spreadsheets at www.riqualitypartners.org by clicking on "HATCh" and then "Workforce." These drill-down tools were originally developed by the authors for their work on Achieving Staff Stability for Better Jobs, Better Care–VT (see Chapter 5). David Johnson of IPRO (New York State's QIO) transformed them into user-friendly, customizable spreadsheets for inclusion in the Staff Stability Toolkit.

Facility Name-	Sample Facility	Date Completed-	01/31/08

This sheet uses general call-in statistics as tracked on the "Call-In Worksheet" to summarize specific trends related to replacement and % of call-ins by shift.

Call-In Statistics

RNs

	# of Call-Ins	
Timely Call-In?	5	71.43%
Shift Replaced?	7	100.00%
Replaced w/ Overtime?	3	42.86%
Replaced w/ Agency?	2	28.57%
Incentive Paid?	2	28.57%
# 1st Shift	3	42.86%
# 2nd Shift	2	28.57%
# 3rd Shift	2	28.57%
Total Call-Ins	7	
Total Scheduled Shifts	30	
Overall Call-In %	23.33%	
Total Call-In Cost	$1,625.30	

Bar chart values:
- Timely Call-In? — 71.43%
- Shift Replaced? — 100.00%
- Replaced w/ Overtime? — 42.86%
- Replaced w/ Agency? — 28.57%
- Incentive Paid? — 28.57%
- # 1st Shift — 42.86%
- # 2nd Shift — 28.57%
- # 3rd Shift — 28.57%

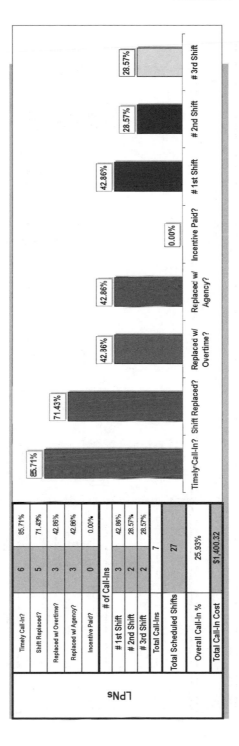

LPNs		
Timely Call-In?	6	85.71%
Shift Replaced?	5	71.43%
Replaced w/ Overtime?	3	42.86%
Replaced w/ Agency?	3	42.86%
Incentive Paid?	0	0.00%
# of Call-Ins		
# 1st Shift	3	42.86%
# 2nd Shift	2	28.57%
# 3rd Shift	2	28.57%
Total Call-Ins	7	
Total Scheduled Shifts	27	
Overall Call-In %	25.93%	
Total Call-In Cost	$1,400.32	

Facility Name-		Sample Facility		Date Completed-	01/31/08

Call-In Statistics

This sheet uses general call-in statistics as tracked on the "Call-In Worksheet" to summarize specific trends related to replacement and % of call-ins by shift.

CNAs		
Timely Call-In?	15	88.24%
Shift Replaced?	12	70.59%
Replaced w/ Overtime?	8	47.06%
Replaced w/ Agency?	4	23.53%
Incentive Paid?	6	35.29%
# of Call-Ins		
# 1st Shift	2	11.76%
# 2nd Shift	10	58.82%
# 3rd Shift	5	29.41%
Total Call-Ins	17	
Total Scheduled Shifts	52	
Overall Call-In %	32.69%	
Total Call-In Cost	$3,569.24	

Bar chart values: Timely Call-In? 88.24%; Shift Replaced? 70.59%; Replaced w/ Overtime? 47.06%; Replaced w/ Agency? 23.53%; Incentive Paid? 35.29%; # 1st Shift 11.76%; # 2nd Shift 58.82%; # 3rd Shift 29.41%

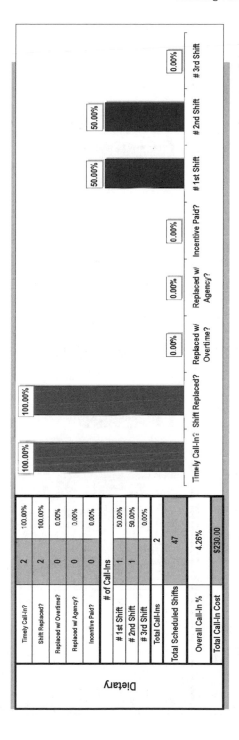

Dietary			
Timely Call-In?	2		100.00%
Shift Replaced?	2		100.00%
Replaced w/ Overtime?	0		0.00%
Replaced w/ Agency?	0		0.00%
Incentive Paid?	0		0.00%
# of Call-Ins			
# 1st Shift	1		50.00%
# 2nd Shift	1		50.00%
# 3rd Shift			0.00%
Total Call-Ins		2	
Total Scheduled Shifts		47	
Overall Call-In %		4.26%	
Total Call-In Cost		$230.00	

Facility Name-	Sample Facility	Date Completed-	01/31/08

Call-In Statistics

This sheet uses general call-in statistics as tracked on the "Call-In Worksheet" to summarize specific trends related to replacement and % of call-ins by shift.

Timely Call-In	%
RNs	71.43%
LPNs	85.71%
CNAs	88.24%
Dietary	100.00%
Maintenance	#DIV/0!
Housekeeping	100.00%
Laundry	100.00%
Rehab Department	100.00%
Office	100.00%
Sample Dept. 1	57.14%
Test Format 3	54.55%
Trial Name 4	100.00%
Check Naming	26.09%
Once Again	0.00%
Twice Again	0.00%

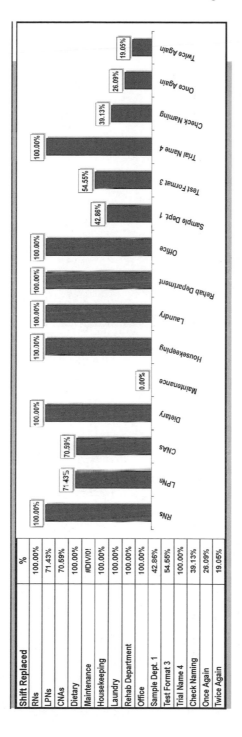

Shift Replaced	%
RNs	100.00%
LPNs	71.43%
CNAs	70.59%
Dietary	100.00%
Maintenance	#DIV/0!
Housekeeping	100.00%
Laundry	100.00%
Rehab Department	100.00%
Office	100.00%
Sample Dept. 1	42.86%
Test Format 3	54.55%
Trial Name 4	100.00%
Check Naming	39.13%
Once Again	26.09%
Twice Again	19.05%

Facility Name-	Sample Facility	Date Completed-	01/31/08

Call-In Statistics

This sheet uses general call-in statistics as tracked on the "Call-In Worksheet" to summarize specific trends related to replacement and % of call-ins by shift.

Replaced w/ Overtime	%
RNs	42.86%
LPNs	42.86%
CNAs	47.06%
Dietary	0.00%
Maintenance	#DIV/0!
Housekeeping	33.33%
Laundry	100.00%
Rehab Department	0.00%
Office	0.00%
Sample Dept. 1	42.86%
Test Format 3	9.09%
Trial Name 4	0.00%
Check Naming	8.70%
Once Again	17.39%
Twice Again	4.76%

Chart values by category:
- RNs: 42.86%
- LPNs: 42.86%
- CNAs: 47.06%
- Dietary: 0.00%
- Maintenance: 0.00%
- Housekeeping: 33.33%
- Laundry: 100.00%
- Rehab Department: 0.00%
- Office: 0.00%
- Sample Dept. 1: 42.86%
- Test Format 3: 9.09%
- Trial Name 4: 0.00%
- Check Naming: 8.70%
- Once Again: 17.39%
- Twice Again: 4.76%

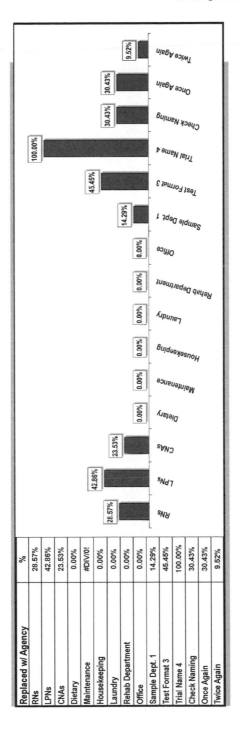

Replaced w/ Agency	%
RNs	28.57%
LPNs	42.86%
CNAs	23.53%
Dietary	0.00%
Maintenance	#DIV/0!
Housekeeping	0.00%
Laundry	0.00%
Rehab Department	0.00%
Office	0.00%
Sample Dept. 1	14.29%
Test Format 3	45.45%
Trial Name 4	100.00%
Check Naming	30.43%
Once Again	30.43%
Twice Again	9.52%

A NOTE ABOUT OUR SOURCES

Work in the field of long-term care is demanding and leaves little time to catch up on current research on good management practices. In this book, as in our work as consultants, we try to distill some of the best information we have come across in these areas for you.

As in our consulting work, we predominantly draw on four sources. Two are from the general field of leadership: *Good to Great*, by Jim Collins, and *The Leadership Challenge*, by Jim Kouzes and Barry Posner. The other two sources are from the field of long-term care: "What a difference management makes!", by the late Susan Eaton, and the findings of My InnerView, the largest database of nursing home staff satisfaction in the country.

In "What a difference management makes!", Eaton describes her research on the practices that successfully prevent turnover in long-term care. Her paper was commissioned by the Centers for Medicare and Medicaid Services and published in 2002 as part of a national study on staffing. Prior to Eaton's research, the conventional wisdom was that turnover and staffing instability in nursing homes was caused by the problems associated with the severe economic disadvantages faced daily by so many of the staff. According to this theory, the instability in the lives of certified nursing assistants (CNAs) inevitably led to instability in the workplace.

Eaton's study addressed the following question: If high turnover stems from instability in the lives of employees, then why do some nursing homes have high turnover rates while others located in the same neighborhood have low rates, even as they all draw from the same group of potential employees?

Eaton studied pairs of homes in three different states, one home with high turnover and the other with low turnover, and identified the management practices that differentiated the two. "A positive chain of leadership," a phrase Eaton coined, captures the essence of her findings: The key determinant of turnover and instability is the leadership practices of the administrator, the director of nursing, and the frontline staff supervisors throughout the facility. Eaton found that low-turnover homes share the following traits:

- They have a positive chain of high-quality leadership throughout the organization.

- They value their staff in policy and practice, word and deed.

- They have basic positive, or "high performance," Human Resource policies for compensation, training, and scheduling.

- They involve staff in designing systems to support individualized care.

Good to Great, Jim Collins's research-based book, lays out what several different companies did to make the move from good to great. We like his commonsense, no-nonsense approach to transforming organizations and see many lessons for long-term care providers. Although many nursing homes provide adequate or good care, consumers are now demanding more. Collins's tips can help your organization become great.

We quote from *The Leadership Challenge* mainly because it is accessible, inspiring, and practical. This evidence-based "field guide to leadership" is a good resource for nursing homes that want to promote and develop leadership among staff at all levels. The authors mix anecdotes with research findings to create an uplifting, easy-to-read resource. They emphasize that leadership is not in our DNA. One of the authors' key findings is that leadership is a skill that can be practiced and learned. They identify five key practices: modeling the way, inspiring a shared vision, challenging the process, enabling others to act, and encouraging the heart. Everyone can become a better leader through conscientious practice. The book helps readers find ways to improve their own leadership and to develop a leadership style that works for them. It is written in such a way that organizational leaders can easily read it together as a team-building activity.

We use information from My Innerview because it contains valuable insights into what motivates nursing home staff and the link between staff satisfaction and care quality. It also makes clear how crucial good management is in creating a stable staff. Asked what would motivate them to recommend their nursing homes to others as a good place to work, staff mentioned three factors above all others: "management cares," "management listens," and "management helps me with job stress."

My InnerView found that when people feel valued and respected, they are more likely to give good care. Facilities with higher employee satisfaction also share the following traits:

- Fewer resident falls

- Fewer residents with pressure ulcers

- Fewer catheterized residents

- Less nurse turnover

- Less CNA and nurse absenteeism

- Higher occupancy rates.

Eaton, Collins, Kouzes, and Posner have all found that the most important thing effective leaders do is to bring out the leadership abilities of their employees. Employees step up when they are valued, encouraged, and helped to grow. Susan Eaton found that homes with low turnover in her study had what she called "a culture of valuing staff." We use insights from these four primary sources throughout our book to amplify strategies for creating a culture of caring and valuing staff within your home. When leaders choose their employees wisely and nurture and support them well, those employees shine, and so too will the organization. In our work, we have learned that leadership development is a key area of need in long-term care and that supportive leadership can make an enormous difference.

INDEX

Page references followed by *f*, *t*, and *b* indicate figures, tables, and boxes, respectively.

Improve Your Leadership and Qualify for CEUs

Long-term care administrators and nurses may receive accredited continuing education units (CEUs) in connection with reading *Meeting the Leadership Challenge in Long-Term Care: What You Do Matters.* The American College of Health Care Administrators (ACHCA) offers the following 5-credit courses:

Leadership: What You Do Matters (5 credits)
Practices for Stability: What You Do Matters (5 credits)
Moving the Flywheel: Getting Traction for Change (5 credits)

ACHCA's self-study programs are a great way to earn CEUs at your own pace. Complete the online test and receive an instant CEU certificate. Visit www.achca.org/index.php/selfstudyprograms for course descriptions and registration information or contact ACHCA by e-mail at education@achca.org or by calling 202-536-5120.